THE LONGEST EMBRACE

A Care Manager's Guide
To Preserving An
Aging Parent's Safety,
Security And Dignity

By Barbara R. Hornby
RN, BSN, PHN, GCM, CCM

Book design by Kathleen Beste
Printed in the United States of America
First printing February, 2015
ISBN 978-0-9862668-0-5

To my Dad,
John Edward Hachten, Jr.

My moral and ethical compass, he inspired me to start my own senior care consulting service and, in his last days, taught me invaluable lessons about the client/professional relationship.

Note on Usage

This book uses "his" to refer to both male and female seniors when speaking in the abstract. This is not especially satisfactory. However, alternatives such as "his or her," "his/her," a shifting use of "his" and "her" or "her" in all instances seem equally unsatisfying. As a result, the author defers to the conventional use of "his."

A Word About NAPGCM

The National Association of Professional Geriatric Care Managers (NAPGCM) is the leading organization for geriatric care managers, and is mentioned several times in *The Longest Embrace*. At press-time, the organization announced it will change its name to the Aging Life Care Association (ALCA), beginning in May 2015, and refer to its members as Aging Life Care Professionals.

TABLE OF CONTENTS

III. PLAYERS IN THE SYSTEM

IV. TOUGH CALLS

Denial is Not an Option

We have entered the age of the longest embrace.

In earlier eras, aging and ailing parents passed away relatively quickly, if no less certainly, often while residing in the home of one or another of their children. Today's elderly tend not to live with their children, nor go quickly into what Dylan Thomas called "that good night." For those with sufficient means and insurance, dying can assume the character of an extended journey through an increasingly alien landscape — beginning in the old family house, augmented by home care attendants.

When home is no longer tenable, the traveler moves for one, two or three years to assisted living, interrupted, unpredictably, by urgent visits to hospitals and rehabilitation clinics. At last, the man or woman, perhaps a hero once in our younger eyes, to whom we remain deeply bound, relocates for as long as five years to one or more nursing homes or dementia facilities before finally resting a short while in hospice.

Diseases that killed quickly now kill slowly; sometimes, not at all. Conditions once dominant only among the very old are now more common, as are the very old. Americans aged 65 now live to an average age of 78.8, the highest average age ever, and those over 90 comprise today's fastest growing demographic group. Multiple afflictions inhabit bodies that earlier would have tolerated only one or two. Alzheimer's disease and other dementias which, were they contagious, would be called epidemic, persist for years.

The modern healthcare system enables the aging to live longer, and pass away more slowly and incrementally than ever before. While many more elderly now live beyond the point at which they can care for themselves, the system also more frequently demands that their grown children manage their medical crises and organize their care as if the very elderly had reverted to a final, incapacitating childhood.

We can only surmise how many adult children find themselves involved in such role reversals. We know, as the boomer population continues to age, their number will increase. Yet, however much it is driven by life-long bonds of love, concern and obligation, the longest embrace — the final stage of a family's filial relationships — can be difficult, distressful and costly, sometimes heartbreakingly so. How many adult children, we might ask, are finding their periods of grieving complete or nearly so by the time their parents actually pass away?

The challenge of the longest embrace is both external and internal. External in that we want to care for those who once cared for us, and assure as best we can that their final years pass as meaningfully and securely as possible. Internal in that we need to do this without damaging our own lives, without blaming ourselves for events beyond our control, harming family relations or going broke. And all while navigating an insanely complex healthcare system with as many pitfalls as promises.

I have held the longest embrace both as the child of a dying father, and professionally as a Geriatric Care Manager and nurse with decades of experience. I have felt the pain, the self-doubt and helplessness children endure watching a parent slowly, inexorably fade. And I have dealt with or seen virtually every type of crisis you are likely to encounter.

I have written this book to share my knowledge and experience — and to let you know you are not alone and that most crises are manageable. Something like a third of all American families are caring for parents or other elderly relatives. Although all will face one or more medical crises, they — and you — probably do not know:

- ❖ What to expect or do in a crisis.
- ❖ The available options.
- ❖ What to do if the parent in crisis doesn't want help or can't assist himself.

❖ How to proceed when other family members have different opinions.

❖ How to turn around a bad situation and preserve your parent's safety and security.

The Longest Embrace will arm you with the information you need. If your father, mother, grandparent, aunt, uncle or other relative is elderly and actively in decline, perhaps in crisis — and you've become wholly or partly responsible — this book is for you. Don't even bother sharing it with your senior. It's not meant for him or her.

It's to help you identify problems, understand the care that's realistically within reach, find assistance, get a handle on costs, and work on solutions. You may feel you're in a complicated, costly, confusing, sometimes lonely place, with a life in the balance, but a great deal of help is actually available if you know where to look and to whom to turn. The following pages will guide you toward practical solutions, and explain how to benefit from and manage a healthcare system that often seems as much adversary as friend.

If you've noticed the alphabet soup after my name, you'll see that in addition to being a registered nurse (RN) and geriatric care manager (GCM), I hold a bachelor of science in nursing (BSN) and am a qualified public health nurse (PHN) and a certified case manager (CCM). I have worked across the broad spectrum of institutions and services the elderly are likely to encounter, including acute care hospitals, a psychiatric ward, a rehabilitation hospital, a public health department, home care agencies, an intermediate care facility, and nursing homes. I helped opened a completely new assisted living facility with a locked dementia wing, and been intimately involved with the licensing, training, assessment, and cost issues that eldercare facilities engage in and deliver.

As a result, I have long been dissatisfied with the huge gaps in care I regularly witnessed the elderly endure. I have seen seniors sent to nursing homes they didn't need to be in. I have seen families ripped off by any number of professionals who were supposed to help. And I have seen seniors' needs and wishes become the least important issues in their care. Fed up with these and similar situations, I established Senior Care Consulting, my own 24-hour, seven-days-a-week geriatric care management company. Assisted by a nurse and a social worker, I learned the business from the ground up, issue by issue and family by family.

I did this because I love the elderly. They possess a treasure trove of wisdom and experience, and the overt lack of concern society too often shows them hugely disturbs me. When I see an aide or a family member disrespect a senior, I try to find a picture of the senior at a younger age to impress upon the callous one that this senior was once young and that we all one day grow old. Age does not slow down for anybody, and we do not all go gently into the night.

I've written *The Longest Embrace* to help you better approach the difficult situations you will face when your mother or father goes into crisis. An early chapter covers the warning signs that a parent's health is beginning to meaningfully decline. The next veers into finances because an understanding of costs and the funds available from family and other private and public resources will influence so many of the decisions that follow.

Subsequent chapters describe the types of care available: what to look for in assisted living and nursing homes; legal, financial and lifestyle specialists you're likely to need or consider; the special, little known role of geriatric care managers; Alzheimer's disease and other forms of dementia; some of the hard questions you will face, like taking away a parent's driving license; and the many things you can do to improve a parent's outlook and prepare for the unexpected. Two things to remember: You are not alone and you are not helpless.

The Longest Embrace cannot address every situation. Healthcare laws and regulations, especially applying to home care programs and assisted living facilities, vary by State. Federal laws and regulations add further complexities. But this book will concentrate your attention on any immediate problem or crisis, and help shape a solution.

Your parent or parents, for example, may resist family attempts to secure help. The senior is in charge of his life, but if a senior is impaired or making poor or unsafe choices, it may be your responsibility to step up and be his advocate. Include him in decisions, but be prepared to present difficult choices he and possibly others in the family may resist. Your goal is to move toward a safer, more fulfilling life for everyone concerned. My goal in *The Longest Embrace* is to help you make the necessary moves in a timely manner, armed with knowledge, confidence, and support.

Part 1

Elders and Their Ills

"Old age ain't no place for sissies."

— *Bette Davis*

CHAPTER 1

My Father and Yours

One day, my father decided to take a bath. He was 87 years old and living by himself in an apartment in Plano, Texas, outside Dallas, near my older sister, Cecelia, who had recently undergone knee replacement surgery. Slowly, Dad pulled the waterproof emergency-alert pendant from around his neck. Carefully, he stepped into the tub and turned on the water. By the time he was found, 10 hours later, he lay covered in blood from his struggle to get out.

I was horrified by the news — terrified both that it signaled the beginning of an inexorable slide in Dad's health and that Cecelia, whom everyone called Peach, and I would be forced into making hard decisions. Dad was fiercely independent and wanted to live alone. He did not want to be a burden to his family. Earlier, he, Peach and I had decided that taking him into either of our homes was not what anybody wanted. At the time, Peach and I both had health issues, and I still had children living at home.

I felt tremendously guilty about this decision, especially since I was a nurse, and also because it meant leaving Peach with the burden of dealing with Dad's daily issues, including paying bills, pouring pills, obtaining groceries, and trying to meet his social needs. At the same time, I was intensely grateful toward Peach for willingly assuming these chores.

None of this was easy, not even what seemed as if it should be simple. Dad would call Peach up to bring over some milk, and she would find several cartons already in his fridge. He was lonely, so Peach and local family members tried to include him in dinners and events. Eventually, he became too ill to even leave his home, so Peach, her husband and daughters tried to bring the family to him. It broke my heart knowing Dad was alone so much, but he was also stubborn and proud. We were all walking

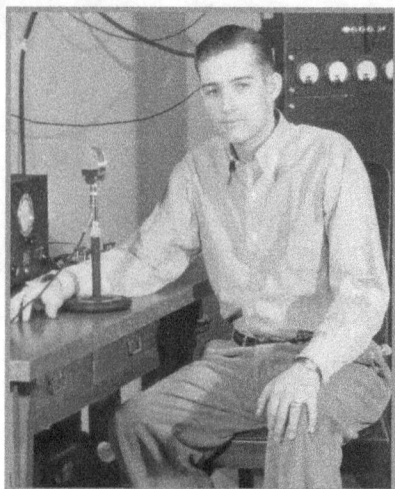

Dad at 17

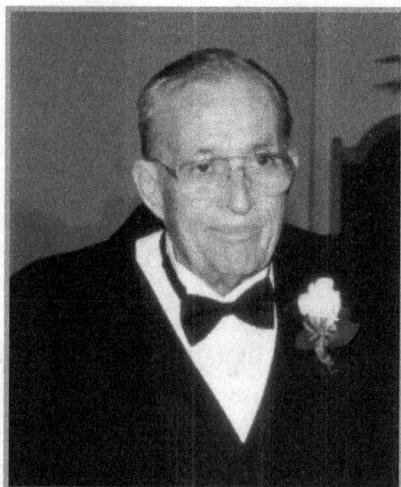

Dad at 79

a very fine line, taking the days one at a time.

But none of us more so than Dad; John Edward Hachten, Jr., officially; known to all as Jack. Born in 1920 in Omaha, Nebraska, Dad was the only child of an Austrian-Irish couple who enjoyed an upper middle class life. Today, Dad might be a Web pioneer. Back then, starting at about age 12, he fell under the spell of ham radio, the era's Internet. He quickly became a proficient operator and built his own equipment. His room looked like Frankenstein's lab, with glowing tubes capable of twinkling the neighbors' lights.

Radio continued to fascinate him, then radar, which he studied and operated for the Navy after completing Officer's Training School. Following World War II, he attended the University of Southern California, and operated a butcher shop, something he knew about as his father, a cattle buyer, had managed a meat packing company back in Omaha.

Later, Dad's love of ham radio, radar and all things with antennas led him into the import-export business, then microwave electronics. Dad never lost his infatuation with radio. He built huge antenna towers beside the family homes in which we lived. Our last family house abutted a 100-foot high tower with a rotating 60-foot beam that allowed Dad to communicate with people all over the world.

Eventually, he started his own business. He was a manufacturer's representative, serving as a liaison between microwave electronics suppliers and technology-based clients that included Hughes Aircraft. A hard worker and a natural salesman, he made it thrive, with two offices in California and much of his business on the East Coast. But he wasn't only a salesman. Our home library always included the Great Books of the Western World, which Dad loved to discuss. He played several musical instruments, tapped Morse Code faster than anyone I've known, threw great parties, and had a huge, rough sense of humor. He was an honest, gentle, amazing man.

Then he grew ill.

At the time, I was running my own business, Senior Care Consulting (SCC), half a continent away in Madison, Connecticut. I was also raising two children and sharing life with a husband who frequently traveled abroad. Still the family naturally turned to me, as an experienced nurse and care manager, to make sense of Dad's health issues.

But I had grown up in California and was living in Connecticut. I knew little to nothing about the senior care resources in faraway Texas. Even though I was afraid I would have to make tough decisions with incomplete information, I knew I would have to do whatever I could to manage Dad's declining health.

Dad was still mentally sharp, but dying slowly and miserably of chronic kidney failure after decades of diabetes and congestive heart failure. To help him live "alone," I had already engaged several homecare workers, one after the other, to assist him in every way possible. Dad disliked them all. (Did I mention he was stubborn?). Finally, we found a great caregiver.

But Dad's fall in the tub showed he had become too ill to remain at home, partly because it was the latest in a long line of incidents. He had diabetes a good part of his life, but remained fairly healthy until he entered his 80's. Then he developed congestive heart and kidney failures. He also experienced anemia, blood pressure problems, glaucoma, and depression. His diabetes soared out of control and, for a long period, he was in and out of the hospital. Each time he returned weaker. And each time there was some 'new' treatment to try or a test that needed to be run, and a new round of rehabilitation just to regain his already poor stamina.

To treat his heart, he was given diuretics that hurt his kidneys. Eventually, we had to decide if he was to die of suffocation from congestive heart failure or of end-stage kidney disease. Based on my experience dealing with both diseases, we decided on the latter, as death from kidney disease is both much slower and more humane.

By "we," I mostly mean Peach and myself. We both had Power of Attorney and made most of the decisions, sometimes without Dad's input but with the larger family's help and support. I even wrote Dad's obituary before he died. Peach selected a funeral home and arranged the military funeral he wanted with burial in a military cemetery outside Dallas. Experience had taught me we would not want to do this right after Dad died.

We needed to get Dad into an assisted living place close to Peach. As an aside, the assisted living model offers promises of trips, socialization, lovely events, and what they flatter themselves by calling "fine dining" with a menu and a wait staff. This is partly a result of the assisted living industry's roots in the hospitality business, not healthcare, in hotels not hospitals. The industry's focus tends to be more on occupancy than healthcare.

After much searching, we settled Dad into one such facility. However, after a few tries, Dad simply refused to sit at a table to eat with people he didn't know, and I can't say I blame him. He was not very sociable since he didn't feel well, and wanted to eat in his room. Yet, every assisted living facility has a mantra about socialization — that it's important to fend off depression, that it creates bonds, keeps residents active, and so on. There's a lot of truth in this. In fact, I had given that same speech many times to strangers. But Dad did not want to play bridge or card games. He didn't want to make new friends. He just did not feel well. And if eating in his room was what he wanted, he should have been able to do so, especially at the prices the facility charged.

But when I tried to have the facility arrange this, I got the lecture about how everything was set up so the seniors would become friends, and that Dad would be gently urged to eat in the dining room and join in. The facility would not even allow a meal tray in a resident's room unless the resident was sick, or willing to pay a hefty additional fee.

To help persuade Dad to accept assisted living, I had told him, "Let's try it in this place for two months, then we'll reconsider." Two months later, Dad became the only one among all my clients and clients' families to ever call my bluff. He could not tolerate eating in the dining room, and the facility would not tolerate his seemingly simple desire to eat alone. So I kept my promise and moved him to a new facility — the only good quality place we could find that tolerated in-room meals. This feature was the open sesame that largely determined Dad's acceptance of our new choice. When he finally made it there, I again made my two-month promise (and prayed).

All along, we were also agonizing over whether Dad would have enough money to stay in a good place, or be able to bring in extra care. I was elected to tell him the costs involved. He was upset, as he wanted to leave his money to his daughters, but we insisted it was his money, and we would use it wisely to keep him comfortable. I firmly believe in this philosophy. Many seniors deprive themselves of a quality life so they can leave more money to the family. Often, the family is counting on it. But the person who earned the money and saved it should be able to use it for his and his spouse's or partner's own end-of-life care and comfort.

Dad seemed to be accepting his new facility, and I had set up a good team of people in his apartment. They gave him insulin, monitored his meds, and helped him in every way. Of course, there were occasional worrisome events. One time, Dad became confused, left the facility and went to the hospital. The ER staff could not figure out what was wrong with him until my niece asked if they had looked at his Medical Alert bracelet or medication list. They had not. Those supposedly foolproof emergency information sources stated he was diabetic and on insulin. The staff checked his blood sugar, which was 22 mg., far below a normal level. He was going into insulin shock, and the hospital missed it.

Still, we thought we finally had a good plan in place. Then, like dominoes, the plan came crashing down. One morning, an aide helping Dad into the shower turned on the spray without testing it, and covered him with freezing water. Dad refused to shower and was labeled "difficult," as if he were a juvenile delinquent.

Then several doctors decided he should have dialysis, which would have prolonged his death, not his life. My family grasped at the dialysis until I talked with the kidney specialist who told me not to have it done because in this particular case Dad would not benefit. Only then did the family realize interventions are sometimes best left untried, and that I was not the new Kevorkian.

The really scary part came when Dad's blood sugars started spiking in the 400-mg. range, about 300 mg. above normal. He was eating almost nothing, so the staff accused him of sneaking in candy (God knows how or from where). I assumed his liver was probably dumping out its glycogen stores, the last reserves of energy in his body.

Fortunately, my niece was in his room the next night. She had called me in Connecticut to ask how she should tell the nurse to treat his hemorrhoids, as Dad was too embarrassed. As we were talking, the diabetes specialty nurse came in to give Dad insulin. I got her on the phone, and asked about his blood sugar. One hundred, said the nurse, who was about to give him a hefty dose of insulin, most likely sending him into insulin shock and forcing him into the hospital — the place he and we did not want him to go unless it was absolutely necessary. Since I was the resident's daughter and had Power of Attorney, I was able to stop the nurse from administering the insulin.

I asked my nurse at SCC to cover my clients and headed for the Lone Star State. I arrived the next day. Dad was tired and weak. We talked a bit, but he did not want to talk about death. I asked for hospice to come in to make him more comfortable. I had to go through two agencies to find one that would come in with specialists who could make him feel better as he lay dying, but not talk about death. The agency honored our wishes and treated him with care and dignity. Death was not mentioned at all through the whole process. We would have gladly talked about it with Dad, but we took his cues when he avoided the topic. He was a brilliant man, and probably suspected what was going on, but we allowed him to determine the topics of conversation.

I talked to the head hospice nurse and we set up a program as soon as I arrived. Hospice ordered the drugs, and the head nurse told us it could be weeks before Dad died, and recommended hiring a sitter so we could go out. We did, but on her very first day, the sitter ripped the diaper off Dad, who did not even need one, and proudly told me he was dry. I had gone over 50 years without knowing what my father looked like in his private area. Now, for no reason, I knew.

I asked the sitter to leave, covered Dad back up, and just sat and talked with him. I looked down, and saw he had stopped breathing. He started again, but he was dead in about two hours. When I went to tell the facility nurse he was actively dying, she told me it couldn't be because hospice had said it wasn't time. Evidently, it was. Fortunately, I was able to make those last minutes count, talking and going over wonderful memories.

I have gone into this detail to demonstrate that even if you think a situation's under control, you need to be prepared for anything. In our case, we thought the assisted living facility would automatically handle certain functions; they didn't. We thought the specialist nurse would recognize when to hold the insulin; she didn't. We trusted the aides to maintain his dignity; they didn't. We had no idea the cost of his care would wipe out so much of his savings, and I had not counted on his dying the very day hospice came in and said it might be weeks. Even though we had Power of Attorney and knew Dad's wishes, there were many issues neither of these could address.

I had long been on the other side of this equation as a professional, but when it came to my dad, so many of the seemingly small, irritating things that compromised his comfort really pissed me off. I will never forget the helpless frustration that compounded the difficult emotions I felt during his last days. Death is unavoidable. Death hastened by clumsiness, neglect, apathy, disdain or incompetence is not. The following pages are my effort to arm you against the slings and arrows of outrageous eldercare.

CHAPTER 2

Is There a Problem?

R ule 1: If you feel there is a problem with an elderly relative for whom you feel responsible, trust your instincts. There probably is.

Rule 2: The problem is usually worse than you realize. Time after time, I have been called by someone who thought a problem probably did not exist, but was checking anyway. Often, an adult child would call to ask if I dealt in "weird" or "unusual" matters.

This would tip me off that the caller did not know how to get help. I would explain that a care manager like myself does almost everything, and often deals with strange, unusual, complicated, messy problems for which simple answers do not exist. And there usually was a problem, a serious one. But by the time many people realize help is needed, they're usually at or approaching a crisis, and scared.

After getting the basics, I would ask the caller such questions as: Why are you calling me now? Did something happen recently — like surgery, a fall, a spouse's death, illness, a stove or oven left on — that changed the way things were? Is there a safety issue? How long have there been problems? Does the doctor know about any of this and what did he do? Is the senior home alone too much? Is dementia coming on? Are family issues interfering with recognizing a problem or getting help?

If you ask the senior in question if he needs help, the answer is usually some variation of "I have lived in this house for 50 years. I have been fine on my own. I don't need anything. I don't want anybody in my house. When the time comes, they will take me out in a box." And seniors have no idea of healthcare costs and often refuse to spend money. They don't realize people do fall and break hips, or that a stroke can sneak up and interfere with the best of plans.

The ideal time to do something is before events spiral out of control and your choices are limited or gone. Life-changing decisions made with little time or knowledge can be a recipe for disaster and impossible to turn around later.

Rule 3: If other people are telling you there is a problem, **listen to them.**

Sometimes well-meaning neighbors, friends or professionals call Adult Protective Services, and suddenly a State agency starts telling you what you have to do. It's much better to head off issues before they rise to this level. If you are not home all the time, you may not know a parent is wandering, driving poorly, cooking dangerously, not making sense or acting in a way other people notice.

I once received a call from a man on the West Coast whose father lived in Connecticut, where I practiced. The father, George, was in his 80's and had some mild dementia, but seemed to be doing fairly well. George had spent most of his career in the New York advertising world and was used to the finer things, including good cocktails, parties, the theater, and a wide circle of friends.

His wife had died a few years earlier, and he had grown depressed. Friends seemed to drift away, and George could appear confused at times and his conversation rambling. The son flew East every few weeks and filled George's pill planner. He had convinced the doctors to arrange George's meds so they would only need to be taken once a day and George could remember to take them. The son also called his father every day, and had him take his pills while they were on the phone, waiting until George had taken them to say good-bye. He thought his plan was foolproof.

But at some point, he began to think that George might not be taking all the pills, so he had a neighbor check. George, it turned out, had never taken any of his pills. Moreover, he was going out several times every night to a restaurant, forgetting he had gone there before. And drinking at night, forgetting he had even had a drink. We learned these details later, after arranging for George to have someone help him at home.

The first time I interviewed George, he was polite, but insistent that he did not need anybody babysitting him. It took hours to convince him he needed a housekeeper for two hours a day to help with cooking, laundry, care of the cat, and anything else I could think of. We settled on a limited schedule, starting with the son's most important issue: taking the medication.

After George became used to the home care and began to enjoy the company, I added more home aides and took his car away. He began taking his meds, stopped going out several times a night, and cut back on his drinking. In short, he thrived.

George died recently of cancer, but the last few years of his life were filled with caring and love. As his caregivers became George's extended family, his depression lifted. One mystery never solved was how a pair of lacy green panties ended up in George's bed one morning, given all his supervision. I still smile when I think about it.

George's care lasted several years, and shows how ambiguously such cases can begin. As a nurse or GCM, one's initial goals approaching such a situation should be to evaluate whether there is a problem, to identify what it encompasses, and then to determine what needs addressing with short and long-term plans. Only at this point does it make sense to assemble the necessary resources.

Ideally, and to the extent possible, the senior should pay for the care, with a trusted child or family member handling the bills. However, if the senior keeps seeing what his care is costing, it almost always causes him to shut out any help.

Often as I wrestled with the task of evaluating whether odd behavior constituted eccentricities or problems, I would step back and try to be as objective as possible. Complete objectivity is impossible in such emotionally fraught situations, but one must make the effort to look at the facts fairly and with unclouded eyes.

If a parent is facing multiple issues, prioritize and move forward. You won't always be able to contain every situation immediately. But standing still and fretting will surely make everything worse, and the longer you wait to seek help, the harder it may be to find.

Let's look at some of the key warning signs:

Storm Warnings

Personal Appearance

- ❖ A parent's clothing looks rumpled or dirty, and his hair greasy and unstyled.
- ❖ There is a smell of body odor, foul breath, feces or urine.
- ❖ The parent wears the same clothes for days on end or is sleeping in his clothes.
- ❖ The parent is not bathing, grooming, brushing his teeth, caring for his dentures or using his hearing aid.
- ❖ The parent is wearing clothing inappropriate for the weather.
- ❖ Clothing and/or shoes do not fit correctly, or are worn in an abnormal way.

Personality and Behavior

- ❖ The parent is missing or forgetting appointments.
- ❖ He is argumentative and picking fights.
- ❖ His facial expression is flat and his word use minimal.
- ❖ His conversational content is not always appropriate.
- ❖ He is leaving the stove on or burning items.
- ❖ He has trouble finding words.
- ❖ His memory is poor, especially his short-term memory.
- ❖ He has memory lapses or blackout periods.
- ❖ He does not want to do anything or leave the house.
- ❖ He is frequently "down in the dumps."
- ❖ He worries excessively.
- ❖ His judgment is impaired.
- ❖ He is not taking prescribed medications or taking them incorrectly.
- ❖ He is denying obvious health problems, like shortness of breath.
- ❖ He repeats himself.
- ❖ He loses items.

- ❖ He uses items inappropriately, such as dialing the remote control.
- ❖ He aimlessly wanders around the house or outside.
- ❖ He gets lost in or just outside his own home (actually, quite common).
- ❖ He is not sleeping, especially at night.
- ❖ He is not eating.
- ❖ Behavior or personality changes are apparent.
- ❖ If driving, he is getting lost, has unexplained dents in the car or even accidents.
- ❖ He makes up stories to cover his memory loss.

Living Space

- ❖ His house is messy and cluttered.
- ❖ Little or no food is in the cupboards or fridge.
- ❖ Food is rotting on top of counters or in the fridge.
- ❖ Bills are not being paid or paid on time.
- ❖ Pets are not being cared for.
- ❖ Clothing and dishes are not being washed.
- ❖ The house is unusually hot or cold.

This is a partial list. In practice, *anything out of the ordinary* should be looked into.

CHAPTER 3

What is the Problem?

I never knew what I would find when I knocked on a door.

But I will never forget one case that might have ended my life. A home care agency asked me to visit a man living in a big house who needed an assessment and a caregiver. I took my nurse partner along on the visit. Fred was peeking out his window as we approached, and asked if we were from the government. After reluctantly letting us in, he insisted on making us tea. He wore a tattered, long-sleeved robe with duct tape wrapped around both feet for shoes.

Inside the house, we confronted a huge hoard everywhere we looked, and the bathroom plumbing didn't work. Fred lit the gas stove, almost igniting his sleeve, then proceeded to look for the tea — while holding a box of it in his hand and wondering what it was. I opened the fridge and found groceries one of his out-of-state daughters had ordered. Fred had no idea what food even was. He soon became agitated, and started talking about the government again. We found out that protective services had been in, but done nothing. We became so worried about Fred's paranoia, we were afraid he might shoot a neighbor or set the house on fire.

We called an emergency psychiatric team, which came out and helped us get Fred to a hospital. The police then searched the house and found a cache of weapons, including a loaded, sawed-off shotgun, right by where we'd been sitting. Fred was medicated, did beautifully, and moved to a locked unit in an assisted living facility where his meds and paranoia could be monitored. Left at home, he would not have taken his meds and could have hurt himself or others.

Determining the nature and extent of problems is more complex than deciding whether there is a problem, and often marks the point at which professional help is sought. Calls from adult children are often vague because they do not understand the nature of the problem they suspect. As a result, I'll ask a lot of basic questions. But once the children start talking, their stories generally unfold.

One woman was giving her dog a week's worth of heart medication every day, which had not hurt the dog only because we caught it in time. When I asked the daughter if her mother had ever wandered out of the house and gotten lost, her expression made me realize this too was a possibility.

One relatively young senior whose care I managed liked to drink glasses of vodka all day long. The family thought he was drinking ice water, and wondered why he kept falling. On my first visit, my client asked his wife for the "usual" in his juice. The "usual" turned out to be alcohol. This got my attention, especially when the husband admitted to boiling water at night without knowing why. After placing him in care, he became ill and had to be hospitalized for pneumonia. Unfortunately, he started aspirating or breathing fluid into his lungs. Nothing could be done except a feeding tube, which the wife wanted since he was still relatively young. But he continued to aspirate even with the tube and died a few weeks later.

Another client, who was living at home with help, told me one day that she was afraid to stay at home anymore, but was reluctant to tell anyone. I grabbed the phone and got her into a preferred facility that same day. Something had changed in her, as she usually would never even leave home.

Initially, I was told these situations were fairly minor, and that's how they looked at first glance. But it became apparent, after observation, that the problems were more serious than the children realized. And my in-depth assessments reflected the more serious conditions my observations revealed.

I usually began an assessment by going out to interview the parent in question, with a family member present to verify details. Few seniors want help. Most resist all attempts to change anything. Many pull the parent card. They tell their children they are fine or to stop butting in, even to go to hell.

This is when a care manager can present herself as a "nurse who knows the doctor," and tell the senior she is there to see how things are (which is true). If you do this on your own, your goal should be to open the discussion in a benign way by telling the senior "I am your advocate and I want to keep you at home, but we have to put some things in place to make you safer." Your parent may barrage you with reasons why he needs nothing, but don't give up.

A professional assessment by a care manager usually includes a comprehensive evaluation of the client's medical, social and psychological condition. It may also include a screening for dementia, depression and behavioral issues. The senior's functional status and self-management skills are evaluated. Physicians' records may also be reviewed, and family input encouraged.

Your work, as a concerned child, will be more basic, but necessary to get the ball rolling. The following lists issues to observe and take notes about. Make as objective an assessment as you can. It will clarify your own thinking and provide a valuable starting point for moving forward.

OBSERVATIONS

Medical

- ❖ What are the parent's physical problems (high blood pressure, congestive heart failure, etc.)?
- ❖ Is anyone monitoring his physical condition, like blood pressure, breathing problems, and weight?
- ❖ How often is a doctor being visited? And for what?
- ❖ Is oxygen being used? Is it being used safely, and for what reason?
- ❖ Does the parent have any allergies or use allergy medications?
- ❖ What medications is he on, and how compliant is he?
- ❖ Does the parent use a pill planner? And who fills it?
- ❖ Is anyone checking to see that meds are taken properly?
- ❖ How is the parent's vision? Are eyeglass prescriptions updated?
- ❖ How is the parent's speech? Clear? Garbled? Slurred?

- ❖ Do dentures fit okay?
- ❖ How is the parent hearing? Does he wear a hearing aid? Can he remove and replace the tiny batteries? Has it been checked lately? Is the TV on too loud?
- ❖ Is the parent suffering from pain anywhere? When? How is it dealt with? Is there use or misuse of pain medication?
- ❖ Are any new medical or psychological symptoms apparent?

Appearance and Environment

- ❖ How is the parent looking? Is he showering and wearing clean clothes? Is his skin looking okay? Does he need help in the shower?
- ❖ What is his living situation? Who is in the house and when?
- ❖ Are piles of newspapers or trash around?
- ❖ What and how is he eating?
- ❖ How easy is the bathroom to use? Does it have or need a grab bar or shower stool?

Behavior and Memory

- ❖ Do you suspect or know of any mental health issues, including depression and anxiety?
- ❖ Are there any signs of dementia, memory problems or increased confusion?
- ❖ Is his behavior sad? Withdrawn? Anxious?
- ❖ Is the parent verbally abusive or actively resisting care?
- ❖ Does the parent feel overwhelmed? Hopeless? Suspicious of others?
- ❖ Does the parent know the date, day of week, his address and names he should know? Can he perform a simple task, like making a cup of tea, and follow simple directions, like "Please put milk in mine"?
- ❖ Is there an alcohol problem? This often goes unnoticed, and is surprisingly frequent.
- ❖ Is there insomnia? Abnormal napping?
- ❖ Is he sleeping all night?

Function and Environment

- ❖ Is there a change in the parent's usual level of functioning?
- ❖ Can the parent make himself and his needs understood?
- ❖ Are there any problems swallowing or choking, especially on liquids?
- ❖ How are bowel and bladder issues? This is a touchy subject, but once you can get the parent talking, he will usually tell you enough. You want to know about any accidents, constipation, diarrhea, and anything else you can find out. A simple bladder infection can cause serious problems, and often presents itself through a changed behavior.
- ❖ Does the parent get around independently? Safely? Does he hold onto furniture while walking? Have there been falls? Can he move onto a toilet without help? Does he need a cane or walker?
- ❖ Is the house set up for safe and easy movement? Are there open pathways and no trip hazards, such as throw rugs and exposed cords?
- ❖ Can stairs be navigated safely?

Higher-Level Tasks and Abilities

- ❖ Can the parent use a telephone? A cell phone? Dial? Call for help?
- ❖ Is he wearing an emergency-alert pendant or wrist button to call for help? And can he use it properly?
- ❖ Who's doing the shopping? Does the inside of the fridge look as it should?
- ❖ Can the parent plan and make meals? What is he eating? Can he safely use the stove?
- ❖ Who's doing the housekeeping? Does the house look clean?
- ❖ Is laundry being done, and is the parent able to do it? Where are the machines? (Hopefully, not in the basement!)
- ❖ How does the parent get around? Is he still driving?
- ❖ Does he have ways to get out or socialize?
- ❖ Who's managing the meds and picking up prescriptions?

- ❖ Is the parent paying bills and managing his finances?
- ❖ Could someone be taking advantage of the parent? Who has access to his money and credit cards? Are funds or bills missing?
- ❖ Is there any involvement by an eldercare attorney? An eldercare attorney is a legal specialist who can give direction to plans, set up a Power of Attorney, and provide senior care advice and services that can save thousands of dollars.
- ❖ Does family live nearby?
- ❖ Are the parent's children on the same page or do they disagree about the situation?

Do not guess about possible impairments to the parent's higher-level abilities. Watch closely and see for yourself.

CHAPTER 4

Alzheimer's and Other Dementias

Seniors are heir to more diseases and conditions than this guide can address. However, one category demands attention for its prevalence, progressive nature and pervasive impact. Alzheimer's disease and other forms of dementia are conditions you, as an adult child, will likely be the first to notice and contend with.

Author Meryl Comer, who spent years caring for two long-time Alzheimer's sufferers, her husband and her mother, called the disease "the dark side of longevity." Like other dementias, Alzheimer's usually arrives slowly and insidiously, allowing seniors to mask its presence for considerable periods. But dementias almost always progress inexorably to a severity that affects every aspect of life and often lasts many years.

Dementia basically means an irreversible loss of the ability to function, especially in the thinking or cognitive areas of the brain. The cause is damage to the brain's nerve cells, or neurons, leading to their death. It may begin with mild memory loss or confusion, then progress to problems in performing everyday activities, odd behavior and impairments in functions like walking and swallowing. Near the end, almost all patients will be bed-bound and require around-the-clock care.

The Alzheimer's Association estimates that someone in the U.S. is coming down with Alzheimer's or another dementia every 67 seconds. Beginning at age 65, the chances of developing dementia double every five years. And at least half of all seniors older than 85 have some form of memory loss or cognitive problem. Most Alzheimer's patients are women, a fact largely explained by women's longer average life spans.

Dementia is a notorious shape-shifter. It may develop slowly or acutely in any of many forms, and for different reasons. It may progress steadily or plateau for long periods, and progress along any number of paths. Some sufferers just fade away, slowly and quietly. Others can be challenging and difficult to deal with. I have had seniors able to stay peacefully at home with varying levels of care throughout their dementias, needing a facility only at the very end, if at all. I have also had clients who could not remain at home because they hallucinated, experienced delusions, grew combative and frightened, and wandered from the house.

One client, Thelma, lived in a beautiful home with her husband. Her several adult children lived nearby, and had been able to cope with Thelma's increasing forgetfulness and need for dressing and grooming assistance. The children rotated bringing meals, staying over, and helping their father care for Thelma. By the time I was called in, Thelma was refusing meds, resisting care, and aimlessly wandering in and out of the house looking for "something." I set up a program for aides to come in and provide structure, stimulation, and a respite for her husband and children.

Suddenly, Thelma's healthy, much younger husband just dropped dead. Everyone assumed he would be the last one standing. Fortunately, Thelma's care was in place. Thelma, herself, seemed mostly unaware of her husband's absence and continued to decline, cognitively and physically, at a slow, steady rate. She stayed at home until the end with 24-hour supervision. She was one of the lucky ones, "lucky" serving of course as a relative term.

Gladys, in contrast, lived with her husband in a pleasant suburban neighborhood surrounded by natural ponds sporting ducks and other wildlife. I entered the picture at a point in her dementia when she did not always recognize her husband and sometimes saw him as a frightening "stranger." She had no cogent speech and strung words and sounds together in what we call a "word salad."

Left alone at times, she would walk from neighbor to neighbor, clutching her purse and looking lost. I tried to bring help into the home, but Gladys was frightened and would push past the person helping her and dart outside (she was physically quite fit). I was concerned about the nearby ponds, wildlife and traffic, to cite a few of the frightening possibilities.

I insisted she needed 24/7 care, but the family refused and stopped my services. Finally, a friend called in the city's protective services. Incredibly, however, the case worker determined Gladys was just fine at home alone. A couple months later, Gladys was in a nursing home. The last time I saw her, she was walking in and out of the rooms, babbling, grabbing items from the nursing station, generally disrupting staff and resident routines, and resisting efforts at redirection to focus her on something more positive.

Recognizing Alzheimer's

Alzheimer's disease is the most common form of dementia. It affects more than five million adults in the U.S., with the vast majority over age 65. But the disease can strike people as early as their 30's. Alzheimer's is progressive and degenerative. Brain cells die and are not replaced. Instead, the brain develops plaques and tangles that prevent its neurotransmitting chemicals from functioning as they should.

In the past, only the biopsy of a dead brain could officially diagnose Alzheimer's presence. Today, brain scans and other tests enable physicians to diagnose Alzheimer's with a greater degree of accuracy, although I think it is often used as a fallback diagnosis if there is uncertainty about the actual condition or type of dementia.

Alzheimer's has no known causes or cures. However, Aricept and other medications in its category can slow Alzheimer's progression in most cases, and other medications can be added for behavior problems.

What Diseases Should Be Ruled Out?

Other problems that may mimic the effects of Alzheimer's include depression, nutritional deficiencies, drug interactions, thyroid problems, Huntington's disease, Parkinson's disease, Pick's Disease, stroke, and other dementias such as Lewy Body dementia, which also mimics Parkinson's disease. In vascular dementia, mini-strokes or hardened and narrowed blood vessels alter the brain's blood flow. An expert, such as a geriatric psychiatrist, is best qualified to give an authoritative evaluation.

My own experience has taught me that vascular dementia, alcohol-induced dementia, and many other dementias seem to progress very differently from Alzheimer's. Some dementias affect memory and judgment, while some affect just one or the other. Non-Alzheimer's dementias tend to plateau, worsen, and plateau again, but usually progress at a slower rate. One exception is Lewy Body, which is now being diagnosed more frequently. It presents Parkinson's-like symptoms along with dementia, and may include delusions, hallucinations, and seizures. It can be very challenging to manage.

Alzheimer's has become a kind of catch-all diagnosis, used so frequently that anyone with a dementia or cognitive loss might be so categorized. This is why, if you are concerned about a parent's memory or judgment, it is vital to have him thoroughly assessed with a protocol that includes blood tests, memory and judgment tests, brain scans, and a psychiatric evaluation. Many large hospitals have centers that do this screening.

Even if a dementia specialist is hard to find, keep looking. Ask your doctor, the parent's doctor, a local hospital or a care manager. The treatment may be very different for a dementia that is not Alzheimer's. I personally have found true Alzheimer's disease and Lewy Body dementia to be more progressive and challenging to manage than other dementias.

ALZHEIMER'S PROGRESS

Alzheimer's disease typically begins with short-term memory loss and a difficulty adjusting to new places or situations. You may also find your parent beginning to have trouble expressing himself and completing tasks. He may often seem confused, and exhibit personality and emotional changes, instances of faulty judgment, repetitive behaviors, decision-making difficulties, and anger and resistance to care.

He may also wander outside his home and become disoriented. Such behaviors sometimes worsen in late afternoons when many seniors end their former "work day" and settle into different routines or find their energy flagging. There may be troubling shadows and uncertainties swirling about as daylight fades into night. As a result, this exacerbated behavioral cluster is called "sundowning."

As Alzheimer's progresses, he will display forgetfulness, and begin to misplace and lose things. Gradually, the memory problems will start to interfere with his abilities. He will grow disoriented about time, place and people. Depression may occur and he will likely deny his failings and attempt to cover up his memory losses, which will be more apparent when he is tired, ill or outside his usual environment.

As his forgetfulness deepens from moderate to severe, he will no longer reliably be able to distinguish time and place. He will lose more things, become fearful, agitated, depressed and/or anxious. Behavioral problems will become more frequent. He may stay up at night, wander outside, pace, act belligerent or become withdrawn. Ironically, his depression may lessen as his awareness of his memory loss decreases.

STAGES OF ALZHEIMER'S

In the early stages of Alzheimer's, a senior can appear normal. His social skills may seem okay, he may not appear to need help, and won't think he needs it. Or he may know he needs help, but is not willing or able to ask for it. He will continue to know his own name and the names of family members, and retain an awareness of past, present, and future. In addition, his driving may seem unsafe. As he moves further into the disease, he may need help selecting clothing to wear, and resist showering. He may grow anxious and suspicious, find adjustments difficult, and start to wander outside his home.

The profiles of other dementias can differ from Alzheimer's in this early stage, but as their severity deepens all generally follow a similar progression. In mid-level dementia, the senior's social graces become questionable. He may revert to a native language, and not want to change his clothing. He will have difficulty recognizing or using common objects, and often be unaware of his surroundings. He will exhibit changes in posture, gait, and balance. He will no longer think about his job or other responsibilities. Abstract thinking will disappear and may be replaced by delusions. He may become suspicious, anxious, and incontinent.

Underlying personality traits usually become more pronounced, which is fine if your dad was a sweetheart and horrible if he was abusive. Once in a while, a senior with dementia undergoes a complete personality change, but this is the exception. More often, existing character traits become more prominent.

By late-stage dementia, a senior will retain no social graces and live largely in his own world. Sometimes, he will automatically recite polite responses, leaving listeners wondering if there is any real understanding. He may take off his clothing, exhibit speech and language problems, and become unable to communicate his own needs. He will have difficulty recognizing loved ones and recognizing or using common objects. He may also lose the ability to walk or even sit up or swallow.

SCREENING FOR DEMENTIA

Diagnosing types of dementia can be tricky.

Remember George, who went out several times a night? He could not remember what he had eaten three seconds earlier, but he remembered my name, that my daughter played the harp, and many other details that amazed me. George stayed at the same cognitive level for years. Even his test scores never really changed. His dementia was labeled Alzheimer's, but it did not follow a typical course. I suspect it was a vascular type worsened by alcohol, not true Alzheimer's.

There are many screening tests for cognition and judgment that you can conduct yourself as a quick way to confirm a growing sense that someone is having problems. The Folstein Mini-Mental examination, once the gold standard, is still used extensively and is readily available online (**www. utmb.edu/psychology/Folstein%20Mini.pdf**).

I developed my own short test, as I like to see how seniors reason things out. Here is the test:

Barbara R. Hornby's Quick Test for Judgment
1. What do you put in a toaster?
2. What does a person do when he has a flat tire?
3. If someone knocks on your door at 2:00 a.m., what do you do?
4. If a smoke detector starts beeping, what do you do?
5. If a paper towel next to the stove catches on fire, what do you do?
6. If you don't have enough money to pay for groceries, what do you do?

7. Who do you call if the power goes out?
8. Who do you call if you see a skunk outside trying to get in?
9. If your milk tastes funny, what do you do?
10. How do you know if your fridge is working?
11. Name as many kinds of farm animals as you can in one minute.
12. Draw a clock, with all the numbers, and showing this time: 10:15.

This is not a hard and fast test, and has no real score. I like it because it indicates how a senior would act in a real-life situation. However, be prepared for offbeat answers. "Swear a lot" was my favorite response to the flat tire question. And one client answered "giraffe" to the farm animal question, arguing the farm could be in Africa. I gave him the point.

THE DANGER OF DENIAL

Like other problems, dementia can go undiagnosed or missed by both families and doctors. I have heard many families insist there was only a "bit" of memory loss, having had no idea how impaired their parents really were. Families sometimes live in its denial. A son taking care of his mother with dementia insisted his mom was fine because she just watched TV all day. When I suggested she could wander out of the house and get lost, he became upset and could not fathom the idea. By coincidence, I arrived for a follow-up visit just after the police had found her wandering on a main street and brought her home. She had no idea how to get home. At that point, the son started to listen.

Frequently, one spouse actively covers up or hides the other's cognitive decline. The danger is the potential this creates for tragic situations. I recall one client, Frances, who had moderate dementia that went undiagnosed until her husband passed away. Once an independent and opinionated woman, Frances "allowed" her husband to start ordering for her in restaurants. Gradually, he also began paying the bills and running the household. Their daughter thought her parents were just being their usual selves, though she noticed her mother was no longer speaking up very often.

After the husband died, it became horribly apparent just how impaired

Frances had become. She had to be placed fairly quickly into a dementia facility. We were all amazed at the elaborate but fragile systems the husband had set in place to keep anyone from finding out how far his wife had deteriorated.

The police once asked me to check on a woman who was skipping like a little girl through a seaside neighborhood. Jesse had been a professional dancer and had no idea she was having problems. She still looked young. However, her speech was incoherent. She talked in a word salad that didn't make any sense. She could not even give me her name. Jesse was functioning on the level of a toddler and was lucky she had not hurt herself. We eventually placed her in a dementia facility, where she convinced several of the elderly ladies to strip naked and jump on the beds.

Even diagnosed, the course of dementia is not always predictable. Eric, for example, was a client with Alzheimer's who deteriorated sharply. Within two years, he went from being able to hold understandable conversations and walk his dog through the woods to a loss of speech and mobility, accompanied by hallucinations, delusions, and agitation.

His wife had researched the disease and expected it would just slow him down. Instead, Eric wandered from the house, took apart the car, almost jumped out of a second story window, and acted frightened and paranoid much of the time. His wife had no choice but to place him in a dementia facility. She had thought she was prepared for anything, until reality hit, and she learned she would have much more than she bargained for.

Dementia victims can also mask their conditions for short periods, appearing lucid and only slightly forgetful. They can even hold it together for a doctor's visit, especially since doctors are often rushed. One of the values of placing an aide in the home is that the caregiver can sometimes see what is really going on. In one case, I learned from a caregiver's report that a dementia-suffering client was being verbally abused by her husband. The husband was making her miserable. I added a fleet of female caregivers around the clock, in part to back off the husband and protect her. She loved it, and remained able to live at home.

Dementia also has side effects you won't read about in medical texts. I was called in once by a daughter to answer questions about her mother, Ruth, who was showing early memory loss. However, I never did an evaluation because the family decided to wait. Since they weren't noticing any significant issues, a delay didn't seem important. A year later, the daughter called, upset that she had not retained me to help her. By then, she had waited too long. In the interim, a crew of con artists had been repeatedly telling her mother she needed to pay them for work they had done.

The work was fictitious. The payments were not, and Ruth never realized she was paying again and again for the same phony jobs. They cleaned out her savings, which were substantial, before the family realized what was going on. Ruth could have later lived a far more comfortable, less uncertain life than she did had the family faced up to her condition when it first became apparent.

The longer you wait to get an assessment and testing, the more likely problems will become unworkable. Early intervention can make the difference in many situations involving dementia.

CHAPTER 5

Dealing with Dementia

Dementia is one of the hardest diseases to deal with because if the person is mobile, he can get into a lot of trouble. Turning on the stove and forgetting, walking out of the house, yelling and refusing care are just a few of the horrors a family may have to face.

Many of my cases over the years involved some kind of dementia, about half of which were probably true Alzheimer's disease. All were devastating to everyone concerned. At first the seniors were usually depressed, then would forget they had dementia, which would often lessen their depressions. Sometimes the hardest parts about dealing with cognitive issues are the adult child's lack of control or containment, and the grief of losing the parent they've always known.

One client, Emma, a lovely woman, was living at home by herself. Her grandson, with whom she had enjoyed a close relationship, moved into the house to watch over her, especially at night. But Emma ceased to always recognize her grandson and became frightened of "the man upstairs," jumping every time she heard a noise. Eventually, she did not recognize the grandson at all, and I had to place Emma in a dementia facility because she was frightened, wandering, and up all night.

Dementia also has a bad habit of foiling the best efforts at its management. No two days or even two hours are the same. I had a senior who regularly wandered through her neighborhood knocking on doors, asking where her house and husband were. Another client, already in assisted living, could not remember to use her walker after a hip fracture. The facility demanded an aide around the clock to prevent falls. To keep costs down, I had to search for a better, more heavily staffed facility that would take her without the extra aides.

Seniors with cognitive impairment can get into big trouble and never know it. The stove, doors to the street, shadows, hallucinations, and scam artists are but a few of the problems that may arise. Seniors may mix up days and nights and do something harmful when no one is watching. Sometimes a secure, locked environment is needed for the senior to succeed. Unfortunately, this often means the situation cannot be controlled at home.

I once took care of a woman, Alicia, with dementia who had a hard-drinking husband. He was dying right before my eyes. I put an aide in the household to keep an eye on the situation, and will never forget the day her husband died. I happened to visit their house just after he passed. Alicia came over to the bed on which he was lying and started calling out his name.

"Bob, Bob, Bob. Wake up!" she said over and over. I told her that Bob had passed away, and she started to cry and get upset. Then, about 10 seconds later, Alicia went back to the bed and started in again with "Bob, Bob, Bob. Wake up!"

This went on until the family could no longer stand it. After Bob's body was removed, I asked hospice to take the bed and all signs of his illness out of the house. The family stayed with Alicia for the night, and she was placed in a dementia facility the next morning. It would have been nice to leave her at home, but she was wandering, confused, frightened, looking for Bob, and needed to be in a very structured environment with constant supervision.

If you should need to place a dementia patient, look for a fairly small facility with trained staff, locked doors to the outside, activities, and a visiting geriatric psychiatrist to help with meds. The facility should also have an internist who comes in, and a sufficient nursing and aide staff. Try to make sure the staff is familiar with the senior's disease, and trained to deal with specific behaviors.

We haven't mentioned medications for dementia-induced behaviors, but there are many and they are varied, with different types of dementia requiring different drugs. The senior in question may even need a carefully assembled cocktail of meds prescribed by an expert, such as a geriatric psychiatrist. Namenda, Ativan, Risperdal, Seroquel, Remeron, Zyprexa, and Celexa are only some of the common names you may hear. Individual seniors can have severe reactions to any of these, so their usage should be closely monitored by a doctor. Seizure medications, such as Depakote, may be prescribed if there are actual seizures or to calm the brain. Ideally, you will want and need an experienced group of professionals to oversee the senior's care and medication.

If you're dealing with a cognitively impaired parent, your job will be hard, but not impossible. Here are some techniques and tips I've learned from decades of dealing with dementia clients. Some may seem obvious or patronizing. They are neither. They are simply appropriate ways to relate to a mentally impaired individual. Use them to make your task easier by learning to deal with dementia-afflicted seniors, whether at home or in a facility, on their level. Patience and flexibility in all situations are mandatory.

BASIC TECHNIQUES

Validate Your Parent's Feelings
- ❖ Offer support and acceptance.
- ❖ Speak to his reality, even if it defies reason, such as waiting for a phone call from a deceased parent. You know it makes no sense, but don't argue.
- ❖ Don't challenge him. Keep him safe and feeling safe.

Reinforce His Tendencies
- ❖ Look for ways to praise him and help him succeed in whatever he's trying to do, as long as it's not unsafe or disruptive.
- ❖ Help make his tasks simple and appropriate.

Distract, Redirect, and Divert

- ❖ Have him try another approach if he grows frustrated, or try changing the subject.
- ❖ Have someone else join you. Try a game or song or take a supervised walk.
- ❖ Present another activity or distraction to interest him in something else.

Change the Environment

- ❖ Move to a different area or change one of his routines or activities.
- ❖ Decrease his stimulation or move to a quieter area.

Get the Person's Attention

- ❖ Wait until your mother or father is looking at you.
- ❖ Speak soothingly and act calmly, regardless of what you're feeling.

Stay Positive

- ❖ Try to eliminate the negatives. Saying "no" all the time only induces frustration.
- ❖ Instead of saying, "Don't do that," tell the senior, "Let's go try this," and do something else.

Speak Simply and Clearly

- ❖ Use short sentences and become comfortable at repeating things, even the same conversation.
- ❖ Don't go into long explanations.

Be Warm and Kind

- ❖ Keep your tone level and avoid showing anger or frustration.
- ❖ Do not use baby talk. It's demeaning to both of you.

Discover the Need

- ❖ Find out if the senior you're with is hungry or tired, in pain, or needs to use the bathroom.

Specific Behaviors

Dressing

- ❖ This can be a battle. Develop a routine, make choices very simple, and provide step-by-step coaching. It helps to find out what a senior's usual routine used to be, then try to mimic it as much as possible.
- ❖ Praise and distract him.

Eating

- ❖ Many issues surface here, such as forgetting to use a utensil or what the utensil is, spilling, and no longer knowing what or how to eat.
- ❖ Serve simple foods, even finger foods.
- ❖ Limit food and utensil choices. Make them as easy as possible.
- ❖ Reduce distractions and allow plenty of time to finish.
- ❖ Offer liquids with solid foods, remind the parent to swallow and drink the liquids. Show him how.
- ❖ Watch for swallowing or choking problems induced by weakened muscles.

Incontinence

- ❖ Make sure no physical cause, like an infection, is present.
- ❖ Establish a toilet routine, even a schedule. Use praise.
- ❖ Eliminate caffeine.
- ❖ Briefs (adult diapers) or pads may be needed, but don't rely on them until you are certain they are needed. Dignity is paramount at every stage.

Anger and Agitation

- ❖ Try not to engage in an argument, which is not always easy. To understand a parent's irritation, look for a physical cause, like fatigue, hallucinations or delusions, or an environmental issue like loud noises or too many people around. Also look at what happened just prior to the change in behavior.

❖ Ask for help if you need it!

❖ Medication may be a consideration. Speak to the doctor.

Wandering from Home

❖ Look for underlying reasons like hunger, a need to use the bathroom, pain or frustration.

❖ Distract the parent, move him away from the door and get him involved in some purposeful activity. Steer him toward a favorite interest.

❖ Provide a safe area in which he can move around when he feels restless.

❖ Manipulate the environment, such as placing a soft stop sign on a door.

Paranoia and Hallucinations

❖ Try to distract him, change the lighting, or get him involved in an activity.

❖ If episodes are frequent, the senior may need medication.

Part 2

Where to Find Care

"Growing old is no more than a bad habit
which a busy man has no time to form."
— *André Maurois*

CHAPTER 6

But First, A Word About Money

We're going to detour briefly to a topic that will come up again and again — the money needed to finance your parent's healthcare. Virtually all healthcare in the United States is provided and insured by for-profit businesses. Even payments from government programs like Medicare, Medicaid, the Affordable Care Act (i.e., Obamacare) and their State-level equivalents, predominantly flow to profit-making enterprises. As a result, your parent's financial profile will most often dictate the type of care you will find accessible or possible. And, though you know good care is expensive, you will be shocked to learn how much.

As noted earlier, the senior should, ideally, pay for the care from his own resources. If at all possible, somebody other than the senior — a trusted child or other family member — should handle and pay the bills. I cannot emphasize enough that if the senior knows exactly what his care is costing he will likely insist it be stopped.

One former client, a fellow in his 90's, once proudly rewarded me with a $50 check. I had just spent several hours, at his daughter's request, visiting him, working up an assessment and setting up a plan for his care. I discovered he had a low blood-oxygen level and a significant respiratory issue. I also took his car away. He had no idea of the cost of my services, but advised me to "charge more and get a better haircut." His daughter, who paid the remaining amount, had not told him the cost of my intervention, fearing he would refuse the visit.

If no one in the family can or will be responsible for the parent's bill payments, get the name of a financial person to help. A specialist, preferably an eldercare attorney, can set things up.

It would be wise, in any case, to see an eldercare attorney as soon as possible to legitimize one or two trusted people to act for the parent with a Power of Attorney (POA). Make sure the POA stipulates one person *or* the other, not *and* the other. This way, only one person needs to sign documents. Do this with an attorney so it is properly prepared. Make sure it is for the individual in question and his specific finances, and covers any decision you think will need to be made, including those for medical care. Having healthcare wishes in writing can ease grief, guilt, and sibling squabbles.

At the same time, put in writing who the parent wants as his healthcare agent, which is usually the POA holder. This can eliminate later arguments among siblings, and move care ahead at a faster pace if needed. If you think trust will be an issue in your case, let the attorney know so he can arrange safeguards.

If there is already fighting or distrust among family members, the parents, outside individuals or anyone else involved, try to have an impartial party handle the money and transparently account for all that needs to be known about how the money will be used. Among my own clients, one family member, often an accountant type, usually handled the money and the parent's bills.

If someone you do not trust is in the equation, insist that a third party oversee the money. And not just anyone, but someone who is bonded, has references and credentials and, preferably, is working with an attorney. You can also have a bank officer handle senior issues, especially if a great deal of money or complicated investments are involved. Banks have fleets of specialists who handle accounting for seniors. Just be cautious. Many scams have been devised to target seniors in vulnerable situations.

Money can also be the root of serious family problems. One day, a daughter who had grown concerned about her mother's living situation called me. Ava, the mother, owned a home, but was renting it out and living, instead, in her car, a local church or a friend's home. The daughter lived in a different State and wanted to know why her mother was not in her own home.

After investigating, I learned a second daughter, local to the area, was renting out Ava's house and keeping the money. How she justified this, I don't know. The two daughters did not speak to each other, and Ava by this time was in a psychiatric unit. I, my nurse partner, and a social worker petitioned the probate court for temporary conservatorship of Ava. The judge was willing to allow this for 60 days so we could study Ava's financial records to find out what was going on.

Two months later, we went back to court for a hearing. The local daughter brought in several character witnesses, and the out-of-state daughter could not attend. Ava said she let her daughter do as she wanted because she loved her and was afraid to upset her. It was agreed Ava needed a permanent conservator to help with decisions. The judge assigned this responsibility to the local daughter, and insisted that Ava go back to her home. However, the judge retained for himself the right to scrutinize how Ava's money was being handled, and ordered periodic updates. We hoped that with the court watching the daughter, further problems would be minimized.

Before you consider your parent's healthcare options, discuss how you and your siblings think about the issue of inheritance. You or a sibling may feel resentful about diminishing your potential inheritance or your parents may want their children to have the money. My philosophy is to be frugal and careful, but spend wisely what is needed to maintain the best possible quality of life.

Whatever the situation, a financial discussion needs to be held as soon as possible. If you know what the big picture entails, you, an eldercare attorney, a bill payer, other family members, and whoever else is involved can use the information to extend resources and better ensure they're wisely applied.

CHAPTER 7

Levels of Care

As age and infirmity progress, seniors journey through a bewildering landscape of institutional care. Beginning by living independently in their own homes, they end, often enough, in hospice. Below is a brief guide to twelve levels of care seniors and their families commonly encounter. Most experience only a few, but all signify significant stages in life's last years, and it's important to understand the differences among them, when each is appropriate, and their approximate costs.

INDEPENDENCE

Seniors able to care for themselves and manage a simple household can continue to reside at home or in an independent senior living center. Typically, such seniors can bathe and groom themselves, change clothing at least once a day, and dress appropriately for the weather. They are able to prepare and maintain balanced diets, shop or arrange for food delivery, pay bills and handle simple bank transactions.

Their health is generally stable, and they can maintain it, in part by taking the correct medications on time and asking for help when needed. Their short and long-term memories are intact, and their judgments sound. They still interact socially, and may attend senior centers for social events or activities. If they live in a senior apartment building that has a dining hall, they should be on time for meals, but also able to prepare food for themselves.

DAY CARE

Day care programs are available at freestanding centers or within assisted living facilities. They can be based on either a medical or a social model, and are usually highly structured. The medically modeled programs should have a nurse and aides in attendance. The nurse can administer meds, and the aides can give showers and perform personal care. Socially based programs generally do not have the capacity to deal with medications or personal care unless they are licensed to do so.

Day care programs are often open mornings to evenings on weekdays, and sometimes on weekends. They frequently provide buses that can accommodate wheelchairs for transportation to and from the program. Their recreational activities may include crafts, memory games, card and board games, and exercises. A meal and snacks are usually part of the program, as well as naps or quiet time.

Requirements differ, but participants generally need to be able to sit for periods of time and follow simple directions. They may be experiencing the early signs of dementia, but their overall health must be stable and present no acute disease processes like pneumonia or the effects of recent surgery. Day programs often work well for seniors who are mostly alone during the day and need some structure and stimulation. Adult children who work often find such care gives them peace of mind during the day.

Day care programs generally charge $10 to $12 per hour, but vary greatly and are rarely covered by insurance. Sometimes a State program will cover the cost. I once suggested to a senior that he go to the day care center to help the program as a volunteer. Only later, after he had grown comfortable there did he realize he was also part of the program. I didn't enjoy this deception, but felt justified because pride often prevents seniors from accepting help unless they feel they are contributing and this senior was part of the program and also volunteering to help.

HOME CARE

Home care agencies bring services directly into seniors' homes, even in assisted living facilities. The agencies come in a vast variety of shapes and sizes, and their services can range from doing laundry to physical therapy. For seniors living relatively independently, they can significantly extend the time before they might need a more institutional level of care. See Chapter 8 for a deeper look at these agencies.

PRIVATE GROUP HOMES

Group homes for the elderly are private establishments in residential communities, and are not available in all States. Group homes are generally small to medium-size structures, and can include private bathrooms. Most offer no medical services, but allow families to bring in home care. Residents must be stable and fairly independent, although early dementia can often be accommodated.

Meals are included and served in a dining room. A manager may oversee the home's operation, and can assist with such tasks as opening medicine bottles and serving food. Costs vary widely, depending on amenities and services, but plan on spending at least $2,000 per month and up. Group homes should not be confused with elderly and handicapped housing, which have income and asset eligibility criteria, and provide no care at all.

ASSISTED LIVING

Assisted living facilities are sprouting up all over. They grew out of the hospitality industry — not healthcare. As a result, they tend to emphasize their dining facilities, grand foyers and varied activities. Initially, they targeted somewhat younger prospects, hoping they would move in and age in place, but historically the facilities have attracted sicker individuals who could no longer stay in their own homes. Most States require that residents be chronic and stable, which means they are free from acute diseases and need no more than moderate assistance with their care.

Assisted living facilities' costly monthly fees generally include restaurant-style meals, housekeeping, van service, activities, recreation programs, an emergency pull-cord or pendant, on-premises nurses and/or aides. The nurses and aides can also provide such medical and personal care services as pouring, dispensing or supervising medications, and bathing and grooming, but usually at extra cost.

Some assisted living facilities offer short-term or respite care, for which families can pay a daily or weekly rate. But practices vary widely. For example, in Connecticut, my State, seniors can have assisted living services come into their apartments, while in Texas seniors must be in a building designated for that purpose.

Some assisted living facilities include dementia units — locked areas with apartments — within their buildings, while some facilities only serve cognitively impaired residents with apartments inside a locked building. This can work well if a married couple's partners are at different cognitive levels. The cost can seem reasonable, but extra fees can significantly increase the cost when you add needed services.

Assisted living is, in any case, generally a transient phase. One rule of thumb states that any resident requiring more than two hours of care a day is too sick for assisted living. And if a senior is too sick or runs out of money, he has to leave — and often has to provide 30 or 60 days notice as well. If an ill senior is to stay in assisted living, the facility can demand the presence of a private aide, sometimes up to 24/7, at the senior's or family's additional expense. Assisted living aides are usually the only staff on duty at night, so if a problem arises, the nurse on call comes in, the family needs to come in or the resident is shipped out by ambulance.

Assisted living, in my experience, works best when medical services, like a primary doctor, come into the building and when nurses are available for more rather than fewer hours. Facilities able to handle dementia cases seem to be the best, since they are structured for exactly that purpose.

Excellent facilities are available, but can be hard to find. Ask around and visit. Look for busy, well-groomed residents and happy staff, and the presence of aides and nurses. Activities and diversions should be standard fare. These places will market you heavily, so keep your cool and ask a lot of questions.

Assisted living facilities run about $5,000 and up per month, with no medical services, and around $6,000 per month and up when nurses and aides are involved. The only kind of insurance that covers this is long-term care insurance, which is also costly. Medicaid is conducting test programs in a few places, but only covers part of the cost and its programs are hard to locate.

I have only found two facilities that call themselves "assisted living" and accept Medicaid. But they are almost impossible to get into because of waiting lists or "suggestions" that a senior pay privately for at least a year until a Medicaid application is approved and kicks in. The level of assistance these facilities offer even seems to fall short of the sparse level traditional assisted living facilities provide. It remains to be seen whether more facilities will begin to accept Medicaid.

CONTINUING CARE RETIREMENT COMMUNITIES (CCRCs)

Continuing care retirement communities are generally for more affluent seniors who plan ahead. Some of the communities are campuses that combine independent houses, assisted living, and long-term (nursing home) care. The senior pays a hefty buy-in fee, often over $100,000, plus a monthly fee as well. The plan is for the seniors to move through the community's different levels as they age.

This type of living is like an insurance policy—seniors can truly age in place, which is good, especially if spouses are at different levels, and are assured a place once the fee is paid. However, if the senior has any dementia or a chronic disease, the CCRC can exclude covering long-term nursing care. Two other problems: CCRCs often lack dementia facilities, and if a senior comes in with a so-called pre-existing condition, including dementia, the community can exclude care for that condition in the contract.

CCRCs are most suitable when a senior really wants to be in a particular place, is in good health or the place is flexible about the issues raised above. CCRCs also often demand the family pay for private care on top of their own cost if they think the senior needs it. After the senior passes on, some CCRCs may return part of the buy-in money to the heirs.

REHABILITATION CENTERS

Rehabilitation facilities come in two flavors — acute and skilled. Acute-care rehabs serve most ages and provide complex, fast-paced interventions to treat the aftermath of events such as accidents, spinal cord and brain injuries, strokes, and multiple fractures. Skilled-care rehabs are for fairly active seniors who can keep pace with a moderately robust therapy schedule, and demonstrate tangible progress over a period ranging from several days to a few weeks. If a senior is not up to a skilled-care rehab's therapy level, he can usually receive less demanding rehab work in a skilled nursing facility, which is often housed within the same structure or next door.

To be covered by most insurance policies, acute-care patients must be strong enough to handle several hours a day of therapy and related activities, a level that's often too much for seniors. For skilled-care rehab centers, most insurance plans, including Medicare, should cover the major costs.

INTERMEDIATE CARE FACILITIES (ICFs)

Intermediate care facilities fill a gap in the poorly defined area between assisted living facilities and nursing homes. ICFs used to be called rest homes with nursing supervision, and many psychiatric and early dementia patients benefited from their level of care. However, they are steadily disappearing, with many converted into nursing homes able to charge more or qualify for higher reimbursements.

Equipped for people with significant health issues, ICFs maintain a nurse onsite at all times along with a team of certified nursing assistants and a visiting M.D. The nurse dispenses medications and performs some treatments. Still, most residents have to be fairly stable, and IVs are not usually allowed. The cost, which includes most healthcare, is around $7,000 and up per month. Medicaid often covers this level of care, including needed physical and speech therapy.

NURSING HOMES OR
SKILLED NURSING FACILITIES (SNFs)

Nursing homes are intended for residents with major healthcare needs who may be in bed or wheelchairs much of the time. Nurses are present constantly, as are nursing assistants, who can maintain IVs and feeding tubes, conduct complicated wound care, and the like.

The facilities offer physical, occupational and speech therapy, and sometimes short-term rehabilitation programs for certain patients, such as those recovering from hip fractures. However, seniors with dementia who are also mobile do not do as well in nursing homes as they may wander in and out of rooms or be disruptive. Since no one wants to see seniors restrained, either physically or by medication, dementia presents a unique problem.

Nursing homes cost about $10,000 and up per month. Medicare covers some short stays, and Medicaid covers long-term costs if the resident meets severe financial requirements. Long-term care insurance may also be used. Sadly, the better facilities have long waiting lists. If a senior wants a particular place, he may have to pay at a rate of $100,000 per year or so for a while, then apply for Medicaid assistance as his funds near exhaustion.

Those searching for a nursing home can log onto www.medicare.gov and compare specific facilities or areas. This will reveal any deficiencies State inspectors have reported, and how serious they are. It's common for a home to have one or two deficiencies, but any place with more than five warrants scrutiny. Medicare.gov can also indicate whether the deficiencies represent paperwork shortcomings or abuse, which is important to know.

GERIATRIC PSYCHIATRIC UNITS

Some hospitals have psychiatric units for seniors with acute problems, generally dealing with psychosis or out of control dementia. If a senior becomes psychotic, combative or unwilling to take meds, he may have to go to an acute unit for a couple of weeks to determine what, if anything, can be done to help. Sometimes, under certain criteria, a senior is "papered" or held against his will for a limited time. Generally, an M.D. can paper a person if he is a danger to himself or others, neglectful of himself, abusive or aggressive to others, or so disabled as to be unable to take care of such basic needs as food and shelter. This is a short-term tactic intended to stabilize the senior, then place him back home or in a suitable facility. Medicare and private insurance usually cover acute stays.

Acute Care Hospitals

Many seniors end up in a traditional hospital on a regular medical-surgical floor for a variety of reasons, including falls. This can be dangerous, especially if the senior has dementia or recently had anesthesia, which tends to clear out very slowly from an elderly body. The senior may become confused and try to get out of bed or present a behavior problem. Some hospitals, if asked, will provide a sitter that will, at no extra cost, sit with a senior and try to keep him calm and safe. If a sitter is not available or busy, the family may have to hire an aide from an agency to just sit with the senior.

When the senior is ready to leave, the hospital's Discharge Coordinator will (hopefully) work with the family in finding a safe discharge to home or facility. Often, however, the coordinator will just hand the family a list of nursing homes or other facilities and tell the family to pick one. It's important to know that you have a right to have the appropriate level of care and, if placement is necessary, some say in the facility and its location.

Hospices

Until recently, hospice was a hushed word signifying immediate death. Now, hospices enter the picture earlier, and provide palliative or comfort care much earlier. Some hospice facilities are like nursing homes or occupy special wings within hospitals.

Hospice teams now even come into private homes. Hospice in the home is like a super homecare agency, with nurses checking frequently and aides coming in a few days a week. At first, the care is not usually around the clock. As death nears, a good agency will provide a nurse all the time, and an aide as needed. Equally important, hospice teams have techniques for dealing with almost any contingency.

The great thing about hospices is that they have nurses and aides, and can administer antibiotics and many other meds, including morphine concentrates that really help people remain comfortable. Many believe that once morphine is started death will be soon and certain. But many seniors facing painful deaths have, with morphine, relaxed, survived longer, and done so more comfortably.

One client, Esther, a 92-year-old woman, was actively dying and the drugs were not working to relax her. As death neared, I held her tightly in my arms. I could feel her heart beating irregularly, almost out of her chest. She was screaming as I was holding onto her. Fortunately, a hospice nurse came in with morphine and, within minutes, Esther relaxed and fell asleep. When her daughter came in, her mom was comfortable.

Esther happened to be the mother of a friend. As we were sitting at Esther's bedside, my friend looked at me and said she knew her mother would not die with us in the room. I no longer question these types of feelings. Esther was sleeping, the hospice nurse was present, and so my friend and I left. Only then did her mother pass away. If people really do have some control over their time of death, I like to believe my dad waited for me to come to Texas before he died.

My own mother died young after a long illness. Afterward, death terrified me until I grew older and began working with seniors. As I gained experience with clients and their families, I witnessed many deaths. I always felt honored if the family wanted me there to comfort and guide them through the process. I also learned that a good hospice team can make the situation much more comfortable for everyone concerned.

Medicare pays for much hospice care as long as certain requirements are met, such as a serious diagnosis and a willingness by the senior to forgo severe life-saving treatments. I know of one pre-hospice program that accepts Medicare, and allows life-saving treatments. But such flexibility is not widespread.

CHAPTER 8

Home Care, the First Line of Defense

Home care is a family's first line of defense against fully institutionalized levels of care.

However, home care agencies come in many flavors. Generally speaking, a home care agency consists of a group of healthcare workers who bring services into a senior's home, be it a house, an apartment or even an assisted living suite. The agency's services can range from doing the senior's laundry and running errands to managing medications, treating disease symptoms, and providing physical therapy. Home care agencies vary as widely as their services, some of which may be specified by State regulatory bodies. If a client is still relatively independent, an agency's intervention can meaningfully extend the time before a more institutional kind of care may be needed.

After hospitalization, seniors are often sent home with a schedule of visits by a full-service home care agency recommended by the hospital's discharge coordinator or social worker. Home care, unlike rehab or a nursing home, does not require the senior to have spent a certain number of days in the hospital, but the agency does have to deliver skilled home care.

In fact, hospitals cannot legally discharge patients unless it is to safe situations. If a senior gets angry and leaves against medical advice, Medicare and other insurance policies may not cover anything. So if your parent wants to leave the hospital in a huff, tell him he may have to pay privately for the entire hospital stay. This always works!

Typically, a home care nurse opens a senior's case by assessing the situation. She sets up a care plan that can include nursing visits, physical or occupational therapy, and an aide to come in a few hours a week to help with personal care. Or she may have a homemaker visit to help with shopping and meals.

Such care is sporadic and meant to deal with acute issues. For instance, if a senior is falling, a home care nurse might suggest ways to make the home itself safer, and a physical therapist could initiate therapy. Often, the need for professional help ends. This can happen for any of several reasons — the senior's problem is resolved, no progress is being made, the family has learned to perform the senior's care or the senior needs to move to an institutional setting. As this triggers the end of home care insurance payments, this is when many families turn to private agencies, or pay the same agency privately to supplement or continue the senior's care at home, if the agency allows it.

Home care agencies come in various shapes and sizes. In the old days, the Visiting Nurse Association was the gold standard for home care. When I was a VNA nurse, I had to wear a uniform and be proficient in numerous medical areas, including complicated medical procedures. Today, any agency can call itself a VNA, as the original VNA lost control of its trade name. As a result, the VNA designation only means an agency that does home visits and employs nurses.

Most States broadly categorize today's home care agencies as Companion and Homemaker Agencies, Registered Aide Agencies, and Registered Skilled Agencies. Let's take a quick look at these and some other types of home care agencies.

COMPANION AND HOMEMAKER AGENCIES

Companion and homemaker agencies are the most basic. They are exactly what the name implies. They do not provide true hands-on care, except sometimes in helping with simple hygiene. They're most useful for keeping up a house, providing meals and company, driving, pet care, shopping and supervising a senior taking care of himself.

While the agencies' aides conduct limited medical oversight, many often perform care beyond simple hygiene so the lines of service can become very blurry. The agencies may be owned and operated by non-medical individuals, and include no supervising nurses. Such agencies often just register as businesses, and so are not overseen by State public health departments.

REGISTERED AIDE AGENCIES

Registered aide agencies, by contrast, meet stringent public health requirements, but usually do not provide nursing care. Each should have a nurse supervising its aides, but not providing actual care. The aides are usually trained as Certified Nursing Assistants (CNAs), indicating they've graduated a course that provides basic training such as taking a blood pressure reading, giving someone a bath, and the like. Most agencies allow CNAs to perform some hands-on care if a nurse is on-call.

REGISTERED SKILLED AGENCIES

Registered skilled agencies represent the highest level of home care. They include nurses; physical, speech and occupational therapists; social workers, aides and, often, other professionals. State health departments oversee and regularly inspect these agencies to ensure compliance with very strict standards.

Two basic types of home care services are those reimbursed by health-care insurance and those paid directly by the senior or his family. Medicare and most private insurance companies usually cover some level of home care as long as a skilled need exists. "Skilled" in this context means tasks a professional must perform, like changing a dressing or providing physical therapy. The senior must be homebound and no longer driving or going out a lot except to medical and other important appointments.

PRIVATE HOME CARE

Families can also hire help privately. If they go through an agency, the agency will provide staff, and replace staff if the worker does not fit in or is sick, though it will be up to you to verify the agency's services includes coverage for absent aides. Agencies usually conduct background checks, are bonded, and handle insurance and tax-withholding issues. They coordinate everything, so let them do the work. You'll be paying for it.

If you hire a private aide yourself — tempting, as it's less expensive than using an agency — you become the aide's employer, and you will have to worry about references, worker compensation insurance, tax withholding, coverage if the aide fails to show up, and many additional concerns. On the other hand, it's often surprisingly inexpensive to hire a payroll service to work out the taxes and withholding, and you can purchase your own worker comp policy. But if you go this route, first protect yourself by checking with an attorney. If you end up the aide's employer, the government can come after you for unemployment insurance fees and other unpleasant issues you may not have considered.

Live-in aides can be hired through an agency or privately, and present the same issues of agency vs. private employment. The laws regulating live-ins vary greatly from State to State; so don't jump into this option without thoroughly checking the local situation. Make sure you know exactly what services will cost, and what they include. And ask about overtime policies.

MULTICULTURAL HOME CARE

Some home care agencies specialize in aides from foreign countries, especially for live-in aides. You will usually need to provide a room for the aide to sleep in and a place to prepare food. However, the senior has to be able to sleep through most of the night, as the aide also has to rest. I often encountered seniors with dementia waking at night and engaging in potentially dangerous activities. In such cases, you will need multiple aides — either three pulling eight-hour shifts or two pulling 12-hour shifts. Sometimes a shift-change aide will come in to help a live-in. Many live-in aides speak English as a second language, which may be confusing to the senior, especially if the accent is heavy or the senior has a bias against workers from other cultures.

AGING IN PLACE PROGRAMS

Every State has some kind of Senior Aging in Place Program that provides limited home care, usually some aides and a nurse on a regular basis. They do not provide 24/7 help, and most are income and asset-based, with qualified seniors permitted only limited funds in the bank, though they may be allowed to have a house and car. The programs can also assist with obtaining Medicaid coverage, which is State-based medical insurance for low-income residents. Look under Senior or Elder Resources on State websites to locate information about such programs in your area.

Now comes the scary part — cost. Companion and homemaker agencies usually charge from around $18 to $25 per hour for an aide. But the more skilled the agency, the greater the cost. Skilled agencies ask $25 or more an hour for an aide, and nurses run around $60 to $100 per hour. Of these amounts, aides receive about $9 to $12 per hour, and nurses about $35.

Privately, you could hire an aide for $15 to $20 an hour, and a nurse for $50 to $100. Live-in aides usually charge around $150 to $300 per 24-hour period, which includes sleeping time. Overtime for the aides, which some States require, can rapidly add to the total bill.

These are all ballpark figures, and vary enormously from State to State, even area to area within a State. Every State has rules covering payment, overtime, live-ins, and more. Some States, for example, allow nurses to be retained as independent contractors, which means they should carry their own liability and worker compensation insurance, comply with the nursing regulations of the States in which they work, and hold a license.

Evaluating Home Care Agencies

Contracting with a home care agency is like hiring an institution to make house calls. You provide the physical facility, but the agency is responsible for the senior's care. Be aware that some agencies, overly eager for clients (competition is fierce), will promise anything to close a sale.

The Agency
❖ Does the agency carry liability insurance?
❖ Is the agency bonded?
❖ How long has the agency been in business?
❖ Does it have references?
❖ Does it handle all the payroll issues? ("Yes" is the preferred response.)

- ❖ Will the staff visit the house to do a free introduction?
- ❖ How does the agency handle a crisis, such as a hurricane or blizzard?
- ❖ How does it handle a medical emergency late at night or on a weekend or holiday?
- ❖ Can the caregivers drive? And are they insured?
- ❖ Do the caregivers drive the senior's car or their own when taking a senior out?
- ❖ How do you get in touch with the agency? And is someone available 24/7?

Medical Support

- ❖ Does the agency make a care plan for everyone to follow?
- ❖ How in-depth is the agency's assessment before care is determined?
- ❖ Will the agency keep a book of notes in the house so you can follow the senior's progress?
- ❖ Is a nurse supervising the aides? Do you have access to her?
- ❖ Can a nurse come in to do nursing functions, such as medication management?
- ❖ What is the agency's licensing, and how many medical staff members does it have?
- ❖ Is the agency required to have nurses on duty and how often?

Aides

- ❖ Are the aides trained in all areas, including dementia?
- ❖ Has the State certified the aides, indicating they've completed the State's training program?
- ❖ Are the aides and nurses covered by worker compensation insurance? And has the agency checked their criminal and credit histories?
- ❖ Does the agency have a dress code for the aides, and set rules for talking on cell phones and other type of appropriate on-duty behavior?

- ❖ Does the agency orient the aides to the seniors they'll be serving?
- ❖ Does the agency guarantee a replacement aide if one doesn't show up?
- ❖ What is the agency's policy if you have a problem with or don't like a particular aide?

Finances

- ❖ What types of reimbursement does the agency take — private pay, long-term care insurance, Medicare, Medicaid?
- ❖ What are the rates? And how do they vary with overtime?
- ❖ Are a minimum number of hours required?
- ❖ Can the contract be ended at any time without penalties? ("Yes" is the preferred response.)

CHAPTER 9

What to Look For in a Facility

Placement is hard work. Few families have any idea how hard until they begin, or are compelled, to look for an institution for an elderly family member no longer able to live at home.

If you're working with a geriatric care manager, she or he will be able to advise you and help you select an appropriate facility. If you're doing this on your own or with another family member, you'll need to visit facilities in person to truly assess what they offer.

The following pages offer a series of checklists to help with this assessment. They include questions to ask, things to look for and beware of, and elements about which you will have to make calculated judgments.

As you examine facilities, do not be afraid to ask questions or talk to staff and residents as well as administrators. Look where you wish, and trust your instincts. If the staff is evasive or reluctant to show you something, be wary. If you leave not knowing how you feel, come back and meet with the social worker or director of nursing — and continue to ask questions. You may need to visit a facility several times before making a decision.

FACILITIES IN GENERAL

This checklist applies to any facility you're considering for placement. Either schedule a visit or, better, drop by unexpectedly. Most reputable places will give you a tour on the spot. Come back again later at lunch or even schedule to eat there if you can.

Overall Appearance

- ❖ Does the facility look and smell clean? Odors of urine, feces or strong disinfectants can be warning signs.
- ❖ Are soiled linens lying around?
- ❖ Are the rooms big enough?
- ❖ Do they have TVs?
- ❖ Are there private rooms?
- ❖ Are there private baths and showers or a shower room?
- ❖ Are there safety measures, like grab bars in the bathroom, pull cords, pendants and call bells?
- ❖ Is the overall atmosphere homey or institutional?
- ❖ Is the kitchen clean?
- ❖ Does the food look good?
- ❖ Are handrails in the hallways?
- ❖ Are fire extinguishers evident?
- ❖ Are lounges available for visiting?

Residents

- ❖ Are the residents up and dressed by 9:00 or 10:00 a.m.?
- ❖ Do the residents appear clean and well groomed?
- ❖ Do they seem alert, content, occupied? Are any smiling?
- ❖ Or do they look lethargic and dazed?
- ❖ Are wheelchairs lined up in the hallway with people just sitting there?
- ❖ Is anyone restrained by a tray, a strap, a vest? Or shoved in a corner?
- ❖ Is the residents' privacy maintained?

Staff

- ❖ Are staff courteous and do they treat residents with dignity?
- ❖ Do the staff, including administrators, know the residents' names?
- ❖ Do staff members wear nametags?

- ❖ Are call bells answered within a couple of minutes?
- ❖ Does the staff include:
  - Physical therapists?
  - Speech and occupational therapists?
  - Psychiatric services?
  - Social workers?
  - Registered nurses?
  - A dietitian?
  - A barber or a hairdresser?
- ❖ What are the social worker's functions? Will she help with Medicaid applications, which are very time-consuming?
- ❖ If RNs are not in the building 24/7, what is the back-up plan?
- ❖ Does a regular medical doctor visit and is he always available?
- ❖ Are podiatry and dental care available, either in-house or by visiting professionals?

The Facility

- ❖ Can residents bring in their own furniture?
- ❖ Are the facility and chief administrator licensed?
- ❖ Is there a sprinkler system? And fire drills?
- ❖ Is an evacuation plan posted? What is the procedure?
- ❖ What activities are available? Are they tailored to residents' needs?
- ❖ Does the meal menu look varied and healthy?
- ❖ Are alternative meals, like vegetarian and kosher, available?
- ❖ How much fresh food do they use?
- ❖ Are there religious services?
- ❖ Is there a residents' council?
- ❖ Is transportation available for appointments?
- ❖ Can the seniors obtain escorts to attend appointments with them?
- ❖ What is the system for wanderers? Are doors locked or alarmed?
- ❖ How are medications handled?

- ❖ How are behavioral issues handled?
- ❖ How many residents suffer some degree of dementia, and how are they treated?
- ❖ Does the staff have training in dementia?
- ❖ What is the plan for handling a senior who becomes very ill or exhibits behavior problems?
- ❖ If you ask, will they show you the State inspection report? (State reports can also be found on the Medicare website.)

Finances

- ❖ What are the facility's fees — all of them — and what do they include?
- ❖ What types of insurance are accepted? And for how much care and how long?
- ❖ What additional or optional services are available? And how much does each cost?

Facilities for Alzheimer's and Other Dementias
In addition to the above, also consider the following:

- ❖ Is the staff trained specifically for working with dementia?
- ❖ Are doors to the outside locked?
- ❖ Are there alarms? Where?
- ❖ Are there places for seniors to wander without disturbing anyone else?
- ❖ Are there enough activities and structure to keep the residents busy?
- ❖ Does a geriatric psychiatrist or group come into the facility?
- ❖ Is an internist available to visit?
- ❖ Is there an outside area accessible from the inside, but locked to prevent escape?
- ❖ Is sufficient staff available at all hours?
- ❖ How are behavior problems handled?
- ❖ What are the policies on using medication?

Keep in mind that moving a parent to a facility can be difficult for anyone. Add dementia and the situation intensifies. Transitioning a senior with dementia into a new environment can raise fears, a sense of disorientation, and other negative feelings and behaviors. Try to bring some familiar items into the new space, with reminders of what the items are. The staff at the facility should be able to capably orient a new resident and make suggestions that ease the transition for your parent, and you.

Part 3

Players in the System

"Few people know how to be old."

— *François de La Rochefoucauld*

CHAPTER 10

Insurers — Public and Private

Senior care insurance is not like a labyrinth, it is a labyrinth. Its endless public and private corridors harbor a seemingly endless array of large institutions, some of which you will likely need to deal with.

MEDICARE

Most seniors carry the Federal government's Medicare coverage or an equivalent program through a private source, such as provided by a public employee or teacher's union. The programs typically cover acute care, such as what a hospital provides, and care in a rehabilitation or nursing home — but only if it involves skilled care, such as nursing functions and physical therapy, and only for a certain number of days per year. Medicare also covers most hospice charges and, for seniors with full coverage, may pay for durable medical equipment like a wheelchair.

As with other kinds of insurance, Medicare programs are littered with "ifs, "ands" and "buts," some of which can be difficult to navigate. For example, a senior moving into a nursing home from an acute setting like a hospital has to meet certain criteria for coverage, such as the number of full days (usually three) for which he has been admitted. And while hospitalization is not usually required to precede home care, Medicare insists the home care involve a skilled need. Home care is also short-term.

Supplemental insurance pays only when Medicare pays, and only helps cover the amount Medicare does not cover. If Medicare does not pay for something, the supplemental insurance will not cover it either. Note that Medicare does not cover long-term stays in nursing homes for custodial care.

Supplemental Medicare plans can be very specific about the types of skilled care they cover. They usually define such care as medical or psychiatric duties that skilled professionals like nurses or physical therapists must perform. The plans also generally require that the care lead to some progress by the patient, some teaching by the caregiver, or some new safety measures. The terminology is very subjective, so if you think a certain care is skilled and the plan doesn't, fight for its coverage.

MEDICARE'S PARTS

Medicare is the linguistic umbrella for a complex cluster of programs a usually conflicted Congress has hammered together over the decades.

Part A helps pay for inpatient stays in a hospital, a nursing facility if there is a skilled need, home healthcare, and hospice.

Part B helps pay for services from doctors and other healthcare professionals, outpatient care, home healthcare, medical equipment, and some preventive services.

Part C combines the benefits and services covered under Parts A and B. It usually adds prescription drug coverage, and may include extra benefits. Operated by Medicare-approved private insurance companies, Part C policies are called Medicare Advantage Plans.

Part D helps cover some of the cost of prescription drugs, and is operated by Medicare-approved private companies. If you are seeking information on drug issues, a pharmacy will often help you pick the best plan, based on the types of prescriptions needed.

Medicare plans vary greatly in their coverage details, and individuals are responsible for making their own best decisions. Fortunately, Medicare offers seniors an opportunity to change plans once a year for a period usually lasting from October through early December. This can be extremely important, and should be considered seriously; **www.medicare.gov** has a fairly good explanation of how this works. If possible, look for an insurance expert specializing in Medicare and related plans, who can tailor a Medicare coverage plan to best meet your parent's needs.

Complicating matters further is Medicare's constantly changing landscape, most recently in response to the Affordable Care Act. Even professionals have trouble keeping up with the changes.

MEDICAID

Medicaid is an income and asset-based federal program run by the States, so each State has different rules. In general, you're not allowed much of either, income or assets. The result is that many seniors or their families find themselves applying for Medicaid coverage only as their private funds dwindle toward zero. Before approving Medicaid coverage, States ask for extensive documentation of all the senior's income and assets, and look back (usually five years) at any transactions it may decide to treat as an improper asset transfer and grounds for denial. As a consequence, Medicaid is neither easy to apply for nor quickly issued. Families are well advised to hire an attorney or a medical application specialist to help with the application, and plan on a process that could last months.

Medicaid, unlike Medicare, covers long-term custodial care in a nursing home, which is an enormous expense. However, seniors going into preferred nursing homes may need to begin with their personal funds (about $100,000 a year); then, when that's nearly gone, apply for Medicaid. It's recommended to apply for Medicaid when about $30,000 is left. There are also bank account thresholds, and rules about keeping a house, a car, and other assets. Some States require virtual impoverishment by seniors as a condition for receiving Medicaid.

PRIVATE INSURANCE

Private insurance policies are available to supplement Medicare, but usually pay only when Medicare pays. If your parent has a private policy in lieu of Medicare (common among teachers and public employees), it is imperative you read the policy carefully to make sure you understand the services or care it covers before making any commitment. It may include some perks Medicare does not cover. More likely, it will deliver less coverage for more senior-oriented needs. The policies vary greatly. If you find one confusing, have an expert examine it. Good luck trying to call most insurers' customer service lines. If I were to count the hours I've spent on endless, unproductive phone loops, I would find time equivalent to a second career.

Long-Term Care Insurance

Long-term policies for custodial care are usually contracted when seniors are younger. They can be quite expensive, even far in advance of their anticipated need. In general, a long-term policy commits to paying a certain amount per day to a facility or home up to a specified maximum amount. The policies usually include a 90-day waiting period before benefits go into effect, and seniors have to meet certain criteria for activating the policy. If you think it is time to activate a policy, contact the company and it will send over a nurse who will assess the extent to which the policy holder has a cognitive deficit or needs help in areas like bathing, walking and dressing. The nurse will send a report to the insurance company, and the company will decide if the policy should start after 90 days or however long its waiting period specifies.

As with so much else in healthcare, expect the byzantine. Many long-term policies are hard to activate, have longer or shorter waiting periods or do not cover home care. Sometimes the waiting period can be met inside a hospital or rehab facility. It's best to obtain a long-term policy before the applicant becomes ill or reaches age 85. Before signing, carefully examine the policy to fully understand its requirements, and enlist an expert as needed. A good one will save you time in reviewing the policy and provide a clearer understanding of its details.

Other Assistance

Many States have assistance programs for seniors, usually living at home, under names like "Elderly Resources," "Area Agency on Aging," and "Waiver Programs." Some are income and asset-based, but whether a senior qualifies can mostly depend on how the information is presented and the forms are completed. This is technical stuff and most families will want to consult a professional in elder finances, such as an attorney or other specialist, to help navigate the documentation. By searching online, you may find many programs that appear to be free, but end up costing money. So be careful and ask a professional whenever possible. Since the rules change almost daily in some areas of assistance, professional guidance has become more important than ever.

State programs often fund an aide at home for several hours a week, and a nurse or case manager to check on the situation. This can fill some huge gaps, but it will not cover around-the-clock care. However, some State programs will help you get Medicaid, which can often provide important supplemental coverage.

Veterans also have some available benefits, but there are, of course, requirements to be met. A specialist in veterans' financial issues is best able to help you determine if a parent qualifies. Often a financial planner will help with this for free, as they cannot legally charge for their help and may be hoping to assist in other financial areas. And an eldercare attorney is always a good resource, even if only to refer you to the most appropriate specialist.

PREPARE TO FIGHT

I learned a valuable lesson about not always accepting an insurance company's denial of coverage from my experience with a client, Jim, who was struck by early-onset Alzheimer's disease while he was still in his 50's. He had worked as an executive for the State and carried private insurance instead of Medicare. He was able to live at home for quite a while with help, but eventually began hallucinating and suffering from delusions and paranoia. He needed to move to a safer environment.

Before the disease, Jim had planned to soon retire and enjoy his life. But Alzheimer's hit hard, and no one could contain him at home, as he would run into the woods. Initially, I had to move him to a locked assisted living facility that did not take his insurance. He stayed there for about five weeks then pushed through an emergency door and escaped.

Following an actual manhunt, he was found wandering the streets. The police took him to the emergency room at a local hospital. However, the hospital had no available psychiatric beds, and no place in the State with an open psychiatric bed would accept his insurance. I was able to get him into a premier Alzheimer's facility, where he has since remained.

This facility was the best, and its skilled unit was well-equipped to handle Jim's difficult presentation of the disease. But it was also very expensive, costing close to $500 per day, which adds up to $15,000 a month and $180,000 a year. Fortunately, Jim had a pension and his wife was still working. They were free of debt and had even saved for this eventuality since Jim's father also suffered early-onset Alzheimer's. Jim had long worried the same might happen to him.

I had been involved with Jim for many years, usually just checking in to see if any behavioral issues had surfaced. I asked to look at his insurance policy, and noticed a clause that said it would only cover 120 days of skilled care per year. This triggered a chain of problems. Because the facility's bills did not specify its care was "skilled," the insurance company denied payment. Even after I insisted the facility clarify its billing, the insurance company again denied payment.

Many letters and phone calls later, it became apparent the insurance company considered the skilled care Jim was receiving as "psychiatric" care that his policy did not cover for the type of facility in which he was living. The company claimed its policy would have covered Jim's care in a different type of facility, albeit one which was not appropriate for him. In denying coverage, it tried to create a distinction between a medical and a psychiatric intervention. The distinction made no sense, common or otherwise, but simply hid behind the exact wording of the policy.

The company's doublespeak persisted even though Jim's care included one-on-one caregivers, nurses monitoring and frequently adjusting his medications, interventions for seizures, camera surveillance, motion alarms, and many other duties only nurses, physicians or other skilled professionals could perform. I fought hard and won full payment for 120 days the first year.

The second year, Jim declined further, but still required skilled care. I appealed the company's denial all the way up to meeting with a board of insurance professionals to argue my case. I won again, and the company paid for a second year. In the end, Jim's private insurance paid for 240 days, but only because I challenged the company's unwillingness to come across and insisted on the plain language of the policy. This did not make Jim any better, but it helped ease the financial burden for his wife.

The lessons: study your insurance policy, get help if needed and, if you're feeling cheated, fight the company's denial. Or find a professional who will fight for you. It took extreme patience and a detailed knowledge of the rules to get Jim his compensation, but he was entitled to it, and it was the right call.

CHAPTER 11

Doctors, Nurses, and Therapists

"All the world's a stage," Shakespeare's Jacques lectures in *As You Like It*, "And all the men and women merely players." In the great play called Senior Healthcare, actors assume a broad variety of roles, from physicians to aides. Sooner or later, you will likely encounter many. Here are some of the key players.

PRIMARY PHYSICIANS

Everyone over age 60 should have a primary physician, generally an internist, who is familiar with the special needs of the older body and mind. Both you, as an adult child, and your parent should be able to have a comfortable, honest relationship with the doctor, and feel open to ask anything. The physician should be looking at all the signs of aging, including all bodily systems, and how they affect the senior. The doctor should also be willing to look over information you bring in and discuss medications.

If you are an adult child, try to accompany your parent or parents to their appointments and make sure you hear what is said. Persuade your parent to sign a release form allowing the doctor or staff to speak to you privately. Emphasize to the parent that if something happens, you will need to be available and empowered to help.

The primary physician should also be able to discuss two main issues with you and the parent: his health wishes, including Do Not Resuscitate (DNR) and/or Do Not Intubate (DNI) orders, if either is what the senior wants, and the issue of driving. Too many M.D.s do not recommend taking away a senior's driving license because it would hurt the individual's feelings, even though the doctor suspects the person should no longer drive. If a doctor can't handle these two topics, how can he address others of significance?

If you and your parent are not having the kind of relationship with the parent's primary physician described above, then change doctors. And don't feel bad or guilty. They work for you, and you have the right to a physician who listens and cares. Find a new doctor who, ideally, has training and experience in geriatrics. Many seniors cling to long-time physicians who are often as old as they, and do not want to upset the status quo.

CONCIERGE CARE

Concierge care by so-called retainer physicians refers to a new private healthcare arrangement that some, primarily affluent, families may find suitable. In concierge practices, the doctor and staff only take on a limited number of patients. This allows them to spend substantially more time with each patient than conventional practices, and the doctor or a nurse may even make house calls. Instead of or in addition to paying for each visit, the patient pays the physician a monthly or annual fee that usually amounts to about $1,500 to $5,000 per year.

However, concierge practices do not usually deal with insurance companies. You're free to submit coverage claims, but you must do this on your own and deal with the insurance companies on your own. This is a key reason why the practices are able to spend more time with the patients. It enables the doctor and staff to focus more on medicine than paperwork. Each concierge practice is different, with services and fees varying widely. Before committing to one, make sure you understand its costs and expectations as they apply to you and the practice.

SPECIALTY PHYSICIANS

Specialty physicians are those to whom primary doctors refer their clients. They include urologists, cardiologists, neurologists, psychiatrists and any other type of physician that deals in a specific area of the body. Each specialist focuses on his area of expertise and should keep the primary doctor updated about any diagnoses and treatment, since coordinating a senior's care is vital to minimizing the risk of overmedication, incorrect medication or confusion.

However, vital as it is, updating and coordinating a parent's treatment among several specialists is a complex, confusing process. It's rarely performed at the level it should be, an issue worsened by the prevalence of incompatible computer programs and the lack of integrated digital records. A family member or a geriatric care manager often has to serve as the connective tissue between specialists and a primary physician. And don't expect the parent to speak up for himself. He either won't, or may become further confused if he tries.

GERIATRIC PSYCHIATRISTS

A geriatric psychiatrist is important to assess such issues as memory loss, cognitive disability and depression. Most critically, the geriatric psychiatrist is trained to detect Alzheimer's disease or other dementias in their earliest stages. Depression is especially common if there is memory loss or after a spouse passes away. I have seen lives turned around when one of these specialists became involved.

Since most geriatric psychiatrists, like any M.D., are usually rushed, bring in notes that detail your observations and concerns. Doctors are not mind readers. They can only take snapshots of their seniors at the times of their visits. They have no way of knowing if a senior's situation is different after he leaves the office unless they are told. So, tell them. More information is better than less.

DISCHARGE COORDINATORS

Discharge coordinators are also known as Discharge Planners, Care Coordinators or any of several similar sounding titles. They are often social workers or nurses, and usually work in facilities like hospitals and nursing homes, where they are responsible for ensuring patients, especially at a hospital, are discharged as soon as possible in a safe manner to a safe location.

As an adult child, you need to establish a relationship with a facility's coordinator to make certain you understand the actual situation.

For example, Medicare covers rehabilitation or skilled care in a nursing home if a qualifying stay has been reached in an acute hospital. However, a senior will sometimes not be admitted, but only observed in a hospital's Emergency Room. In such cases, which can last several days, the time won't count toward Medicare days, and the senior will be billed.

Always ask the coordinator if the qualifying stay has met Medicare's requirements. At some point, the coordinator may hand you a list of nursing homes or home care agencies, and say something like "pick one now." The coordinator may expect you to digest everything and answer immediately, but you have the right to deliberate, look over the list, select what you want within reason, or ask to see someone else from the Discharge Planning Office to help you. Geriatric care managers, who are experienced at working with discharge planners, are especially helpful at this point.

Geriatric Care Managers

Geriatric care managers specialize in helping seniors and their families identify and assess problems, find and implement solutions, and create the best possible resolution for all concerned. Their main goal is quality of life for seniors and their families. Their role has become so central to good senior care that Chapter 12 discusses this specialty in depth.

Nurses

Nurses are omnipresent throughout the healthcare continuum. Most are RNs with training in many areas. Those working with seniors should have geriatric experience. Licensed practical nurses (LPNs) can perform most of the duties of an RN, but often RNs have to supervise. Advanced Practice Nurses (APRNs) and Physician Assistants (PAs) can prescribe medication, and often step in for a doctor. They always work under the overall supervision of a physician, although APRNs are moving toward more independence.

Nurses can assist with care and interventions, and should show seniors compassion and respect. They should be well dressed and groomed, wash their hands before touching seniors, and feel comfortable dealing with whatever physical or mental problems may be going on. They should have support and back-up from their agencies or facilities, know how to talk with family members, be able to put seniors at ease, and be familiar enough with dementia to identify and deal with it.

Nurses also serve as the eyes and ears of physicians, and should be expected to use their professionally educated brains. I have seen instances of clients severely over-medicated in facilities and at home, with the nurse blaming the doctor for writing the order. A truly effective nurse should always put the patient first. If she suspects a medication's dose may be incorrect or its effects harmful or inappropriate, it is up to her to confront the prescribing doctor and, if necessary, refuse to administer the medication or treatment until the situation is resolved.

It is very important to develop a relationship with the nurse in any setting. But, as in any profession, there are good and not-so-good ones. If you don't like your nurse, ask for another.

SOCIAL WORKERS

Social workers are sprinkled across the healthcare spectrum. They can serve as counselors, discharge coordinators, benefit specialists or any number of other roles. They may or may not have a degree or a license. Non-licensed social workers often work under the supervision of a licensed and certified social worker.

Social workers should be able to help deal with family discord, determine safe home situations, order equipment, cope with Medicaid applications, and sniff out benefits of which seniors (such as veterans) and their families may be unaware. While there are good and mediocre social workers, expect those with whom you deal to be comfortable working with seniors, dementia, the medical system, and families in distress. If you're displeased with your social worker, ask for another.

AIDES OR NURSE'S AIDES

Aides comprise a very diverse group of caregivers in terms of age, experience, personality, ethnicity, ability, and their comfort level working with sick and/or demented seniors. In selecting an aide, look for a good fit, but be patient. Some relationships between seniors and aides start rocky but turn out well given time. Aides can serve as companions or homemakers and more, especially if State-certified and supervised by a nurse. Their focus should be on the care and dignity of the senior.

Aides should always dress neatly, groom appropriately, and use cell phones only for emergencies. They can wear scrubs or street clothes in the home — whatever you are comfortable with. Some agencies require a uniform, but you, the customer, can usually request what you would like an aide to wear. Some seniors like the crisp look of scrubs, while others are embarrassed to be seen in public with an obvious caregiver.

States mandate what certified aides can do, but you should carefully scrutinize every aide. I have sometimes encountered cases of theft and manipulation of seniors. On the other hand, when you deal with an excellent aide, reward her with praise and compliments.

Aides who have cared for a client over a long period of time often feel a sense of ownership toward the client. Some of this attitude is good; you want an aide to feel responsible and accountable. However, I have seen many an aide challenge the wishes of the supervising nurse or family, believing her way to be the only right way. This is simply inappropriate. The aide works for the client and his family, and needs to take direction. If this becomes an issue, speak to the aide directly or to her supervisor. But try to do it tactfully. You don't want an angry or demoralized aide taking care of a loved one. If you remain uncomfortable about the situation, replace the aide.

PHYSICAL THERAPISTS

A good physical therapist can make a huge difference in a parent's life. A therapist can assist with walking, strength training, moving around more safely, and modifying the home. A senior can lose all his strength just by resting in bed for a day or two, and a weak or de-conditioned senior is a fall waiting to happen.

OCCUPATIONAL THERAPISTS

Occupational therapists concentrate on the fine muscles and activities needed for daily living. They help seniors perform and improve such tasks as cooking, eating, grooming, dressing, and brushing teeth. They also can suggest home modifications.

Speech Therapists

Helping seniors regain their speech is only one aspect of what speech therapists do. For example, they can also perform tests for swallowing, necessary since some seniors swallow incorrectly, leaving tiny amounts of food or fluid to end up in their lungs, causing aspiration pneumonia. This is often an insidious cause of death and more common than most realize. Speech therapists offer exercises to correct this, and can also recommend modifying the consistency of a senior's food, or even his food choices, if it will make a difference. A therapist may also refer the senior for more extensive testing, including X-rays taken after swallowing an imaging contrast medium, such as barium.

Podiatrists

Podiatrists deal with feet, and provide seniors with necessary services, especially seniors with diabetes, because of which cuts and wounds heal more slowly. Diabetes can also cause neuropathy that may blunt feelings of pain, sometimes leading to horrific sores and infections.

A senior should see a podiatrist at least every few months for a complete foot assessment, nail trimming, and any required interventions. The podiatrist should be patient and comfortable with seniors. He should not only look at a senior's feet, but also evaluate his gait and footwear, and offer suggestions.

In some areas, podiatrists and podiatry nurses are available to make house calls to seniors' homes. They can handle almost anything, and refer seniors to podiatry offices for serious problems. The nurses tend not to accept insurance, but are relatively inexpensive, and the seniors I've known who used them were grateful every time.

A word about toenails. Cutting difficult ones can seem to require only the right clipper. But families don't have them. In addition, seniors' nails can grow into the skin in ways that make trimming them impossible for amateurs. And if a senior has dementia, he needs to be handled carefully by a seasoned professional. Podiatrists have custom grinders, sanders, and scissors made for difficult toenails. And they know how to use them. Let them.

DENTISTS

All seniors need dentistry. The reasons are legion — rotting teeth, bridges, dentures, gum problems, discomfort, embarrassment and much more. Find a dentist who's comfortable with seniors, including those with dementia. Be completely frank with the dentist and his staff about any issues, bearing in mind the senior may not speak up. It is usually best if a family member or care manager goes into the office with the senior, as there may be follow-up requirements and additional procedures.

A few dentists make house calls, but without their equipment, making it difficult to perform most procedures. If a very expensive intervention is recommended, ask if there are alternatives and if the procedure is necessary. Sometimes, a dentist will spend time and charge a small fortune to save a rotten tooth or recommend an expensive implant for someone very elderly. Often it will be more practical to just have a bad tooth pulled, solving a problem at minimal cost.

CHAPTER 12

Geriatric Care Managers

Geriatric care managers (GCMs) warrant a more in-depth treatment. Little known outside healthcare circles, they can play an important, even critical, role in determining the course of a senior's care. However, few seniors or their adult children are aware of GCMs and their capabilities, especially prior to a crisis. Simply put, geriatric care managers specialize in assisting seniors and their families in identifying problems, finding and implementing solutions, and creating the best possible outcomes for all involved. A GCM's primary goal is quality of life for the senior and the senior's family. And if a family lives in a different State than the senior's State, the GCM is uniquely positioned to step in to oversee a senior's care.

GCMs can be nurses, doctors, social workers or other professionals who meet the requirements for GCM certification, which is overseen by the National Association of Professional Geriatric Care Managers (www. caremanager.org). The group's website explains what a GCM does, its code of ethics, and how to find one in your area. It also includes a directory with information about individual GCMs.

I happen to be a nurse, and was already practicing Care Management before I knew the NAPGCM existed, an indication of the profession's obscurity. Once I learned about the organization, I immediately became a member. All GCMs have their own way of conducting their practices. My motto was to do whatever it took. As a nurse, I was qualified to provide care as well as manage it. This led me to offer seniors and their families a broad menu of services.

My services almost always began with a consultation. This entailed a one-time visit with the senior and/or family members to introduce them to what a Geriatric Care Manager has to offer, and to gain a preliminary overview of the situation. During the consultation, I would evaluate the senior's condition, functional level, living situation, and note any special challenges. I would also answer questions about locally based services, facilities or resources that I might recommend.

Following the consultation, I would usually proceed toward making a fuller assessment of the situation. By assessment, I mean a comprehensive, in-depth evaluation of the medical, social and psychological situation of the senior client (usually a parent).

The assessment might include:

- ❖ A phone interview with the parent or a family member.
- ❖ An onsite assessment of the parent's living situation and any medical, social, psychological issues.
- ❖ Screening for dementia, depression and behavioral issues.
- ❖ A determination of the parent's functional status, daily living abilities, and self-management skills.
- ❖ A medical history review, including requests to the parent's primary M.D. and/or other caregivers for additional information.
- ❖ A screening of the parent's home or facility for safety issues.
- ❖ A review with the parent and/or family members of my findings and suggestions for services, care, equipment, home modifications, referrals, and, if needed, placement.
- ❖ A written, detailed report of my assessment and recommendations.
- ❖ Initial referrals for services, a facility or equipment.

After an assessment, I would remain available to assist with coordinating and managing the parent's care. My additional services included:

- ❖ Counseling the parent and/or his family.
- ❖ Serving as a liaison to other caregivers and professionals.
- ❖ Explaining to families the different types and levels of senior care, the pluses and drawbacks of each, and the costs involved.

- ❖ Monitoring the parent at home or in a facility through daily, weekly or occasional visits.
- ❖ Performing basic nursing functions in coordination with a parent's physician.
- ❖ Serving as an advocate and liaison for hospitalized parents.
- ❖ Reviewing the parent's medical chart and coordinating services for a hospitalized parent.
- ❖ Accompanying parents to doctor, attorney or other appointments.
- ❖ Accompanying parents on airplanes or other transit modes to manage behavioral or physical issues.
- ❖ Providing in-depth information, including statistics and deficiencies, about services and facilities.
- ❖ Making referrals to M.D.s, specialists, programs or facilities, and dealing with their sales and marketing personnel.
- ❖ Providing referrals to attorneys specializing in eldercare, and following up as needed.
- ❖ Dealing with the specific needs of parents with dementia and the families supporting them.
- ❖ Training and monitoring staff providing services at home or in a facility.
- ❖ Moving a parent to a more appropriate facility if needed.
- ❖ Assisting a parent in adjusting to a new program or facility.
- ❖ Attending care plan meetings as the parent's advocate.
- ❖ Meeting with family members, individually or as a group, to overcome resistance and help everyone work toward the same goal. Families frequently need help in moving forward.
- ❖ Meeting with and maintaining positive relationships with police or adult protective services, if needed.
- ❖ Assisting with insurance issues, such as long-term care or veteran benefits.
- ❖ Assisting with end of life care, such as administering medication and care in the home.
- ❖ Preparing probate court documents and testimony.

In my own practice, I typically began a new case with a phone call from a concerned family member. One or more phone conversations (at no cost) usually allowed me to get an idea of what was going on and helped the caller to understand my services. If we moved forward, the senior, or more often a responsible family member, would sign a contract, supply certain demographic information, and sign a health information release form. I would send the release form to the senior's doctor with a questionnaire. I would also set up an extensive assessment with the senior and family members, visit the senior's house and spend at least two to four hours getting to the root of the situation. If the family had a Power of Attorney already in place, this part of the process always proceeded more quickly and easily.

During my initial visit, I would find out all medical problems, and assess memory issues. I would use a Folstein Mini-mental test (available online at **www.utmb.edu/psychology/Folstein%20Mini.pdf**), and my own test for judgment (see Chapter 4). I would review the senior's medications, and assess the safety of the home. Often, I would speak with additional family members to get a more complete picture.

I would then write a report stating my observations, my concerns and my suggestions for solutions. I would send the report to the senior's physician and give a copy to the senior and his family. At this point, the senior and his family could continue to retain my services or use my information and go ahead on their own.

Usually, I developed continuing relationships with the seniors I assessed, visiting regularly to monitor our interventions or provide care, and to keep in the loop with the family. In most cases, the senior's adult child would pay me using the senior's funds.

I always maintained access to the community's senior care resources. Since I knew my clients' financial profiles, I was able to tailor my plans to what they could afford. I always tried to deliver the best for the least amount of money, as healthcare is expensive. If there was a service Medicare would cover, such as a visiting nurse, I would exhaust that first or augment it. And I or my office were always on call, enabling me to go quickly to a senior's home to assess a developing situation and, hopefully, avoid a hospitalization.

One of the best roles a GCM can play is as an objective professional. A GCM is not a senior's adult child or friend. I always told the senior I was a nurse who was there to help, that my goal was to keep him at home and safe, and that I would work with his doctor. No senior ever threw me out or even asked much beyond this. I also convened family meetings, helped settle family squabbles, advocated for the senior, and played the tough guy to seniors who resisted needed care. It's too easy for a senior to tell the children to back off.

You can locate a good GCM by starting with the NAPGCM website (www.caremanager.org), and then interviewing individuals in whom you're interested. Ask specific questions and don't be afraid to ask about experience. You need to feel comfortable with your Care Manager.

I generally charged $100 per hour during business hours, $200 an hour for nights, weekends and holidays, and half the hourly fee for travel. This may seem like a lot, but a good GCM can save thousands in the long run. And I did not usually charge for phone conversations with families as long as they did not take all my time. I wanted the families to feel comfortable enough to ask me anything. Many GCM's structure their fees differently as seniors and situations vary so widely.

CHAPTER 13

Lawyers, Managers, and Consultants

Continuing our tour of the healthcare landscape, we come to the non-medical side of the community, which is populated by a broad array of specialized professionals. Here are some key players and the services they offer.

ATTORNEYS

Most of us cringe at the thought of going to a lawyer, but attorneys can help make vital decisions that allow seniors and families to deploy their assets in the best possible way. However, the most important point I can emphasize here is to find an attorney that specializes in eldercare.

Eldercare attorneys understand estate planning and ways to protect or enhance assets. They're familiar with Medicaid laws, "special needs" trusts, and options for maximizing income. Some have begun to offer so-called Lifecare Planning, which is designed to comprehensively address the financial issues and needs of seniors and their families, as well as their living situations.

Eldercare attorneys can advise about healthcare wishes and reverse mortgages. They can process Power of Attorney appointments to designated family members, and customize POAs to give, for example, one person authority over issues like healthcare, and another person authority over financial issues. Eldercare attorneys can also handle conservatorships, which occur when a senior can no longer make safe decisions and a family member, friend or court-appointee takes charge of personal and financial issues.

The attorney is, in addition, the go-to person for mediating certain sticky family issues, especially if family or probate court is involved, as in a conservatorship. With mediation a recognized service, some attorneys now specialize in Elder Mediation. This is a wonderful development. I have observed some ugly family confrontations over old wounds triggered by sibling rivalries and resentments. Trained mediators can play vital roles in resolving such situations as much as possible and moving the seniors and families forward.

Many eldercare attorneys have staff to assist in applying for Medicaid, which is very complicated. Each State's application is different, but most include a multi-year look-back period for spending. This allows a State to disqualify Medicaid claims if it decides a senior has improperly given away, shed, or concealed money or other assets in the recent past.

In such cases, the State will deny Medicaid, make the senior wait for it or apply a huge penalty. This can be extremely stressful. If the senior or his family is running out of money, he needs the Medicaid coverage in a timely manner, especially if his placement in a nursing home depends on private funds that no longer exist.

I remember one client who had applied for Medicaid and owned a piece of property the family had forgotten about. It was an inaccessible and, therefore, unsalable lot, but the State still put a lien on it. The daughter finally sold it to a neighbor for peanuts just to get the State and her father's nursing facility, both of which were demanding the proceeds of a forced sale, off her back.

In looking for an eldercare attorney, ask around for references. Most attorneys will provide a free consultation to discuss options. Retain a qualified attorney with experience, and be aware many lawyers who are not eldercare specialists will say they are. Sometimes, a senior will want to a use real estate or other attorney he has known for decades for eldercare guidance. This is usually not a good idea.

FINANCE AND ESTATE MANAGERS

Finance and estate managers tend to be accountants or money managers. They can help organize finances, pay bills, and coordinate house expenses. Make sure any you use is licensed and bonded, and provides frequent updates. Some attorneys offer finance management through their offices.

Large banks usually have staff that can handle senior finances. Ask around for referrals, then check that person's qualifications and ability to deal with a senior directly.

Seniors can be very unwilling to part with any money, and suspicious of a stranger handling it. Don't blame them for this. The senior needs to trust and feel comfortable with the money person, and so do you. It's also imperative the manager have an above average amount of patience. Many times I have wanted to scream while a senior went over every word and number in a financial report, obsessing over each and every item. The manager will need to go over everything with the senior and his family, and also be able to manage (at least up to a point) any family discord. Nothing compares with money in bringing out the more argumentative inclinations of family members.

Benefit Consultants

If you need more help than finance and estate managers offer, look into working with a designated benefit consultant who can deal with Veteran Administration benefits and other less familiar sources of reimbursement. For example, some States offer programs for respite care, allowing seniors, especially ones suffering from dementia, to stay in assisted living for short periods of time to give the family some needed rest. Reverse mortgages are gaining in popularity, but you'll need a professional to guide you through their many risks.

Employee Assistance Programs

Larger companies often have programs to help employees with senior issues, having realized that employees dealing with the difficulties aging parents present can lead to absences or decreased attention at work. At the least, such assistance programs will be able to offer names and contact information for care managers or other essential resources. Ask your company's Human Resources department if a program is available.

Adult or Elderly Protective Services

Adult or elderly protective services can be brought into the picture by anybody, neighbors included, who reports a safety concern. Protective service employees work for the State, and can make legally enforceable demands as severe as nursing home placement.

I remember one couple, in particular, whose daughter had to call in protective services. The husband, a non-English speaker from a foreign culture, was highly agitated and exhibiting memory loss. His wife was very ill, and they fought almost constantly. Living mostly in one room of their house, they were no longer able to safely cook for themselves. They suffered from falls, and were attempting to drive. The daughter was desperately trying to help, but had reached her limit.

I had the couple placed in an assisted living dementia facility so their house could be cleaned out and made safer. We hoped to get them back home and provided with care. However one day, the husband called a car rental agency to have a car delivered to him at the dementia facility. We caught it just in time. But the couple made such a scene the facility "encouraged" them to leave.

I brought in an interpreter for the husband. We tried to keep the couple secure for two more weeks, but they would have none of it. They returned home before the house was ready, and more than one person called protective services. The agency came in, insisted they have full-time home care, and monitored the situation.

I still wonder what the rental agency delivering the car to a locked dementia facility thought it was doing.

CHAPTER 14

Lifestylers

With so many medical, safety and financial problems to consider, preserving a senior's quality of life often takes a back seat to more urgent issues. But quality of life is important. Fortunately, a universe of specialists exists to help seniors pass their final years with a little more comfort and dignity than they otherwise might.

Many of these individuals work as freelancers or independent contractors. Some provide services that are unknown to seniors and their families until needed. Here are a few of the more frequently used specialties.

PROFESSIONAL ORGANIZERS

Many professional organizers specialize in working with seniors. They cover everything from downsizing a home or apartment and helping seniors decide what to keep, to bringing in appraisers and arranging actual moves. They also deal with hoarding issues. I have worked with many organizers, and the best were not only personable and hard-working, but they made their seniors feel like they had an advocate.

Downsizing from a home to assisted living can be very depressing, and good professional organizers try to make the transition a smooth one. Families often get stuck helping seniors move, especially if there is a home full of memories. Organizers can prioritize the process in ways that help seniors make smart choices about what to take or leave. Make sure anyone you retain is bonded and insured, and ask for references.

PET SITTERS

Many home care agencies perform pet sitting along with human health-care. Aides generally like caring for animals, and fold it into their regular duties. If this is not the case with your agency, freelance pet sitters, walkers and trainers are readily available. Local veterinarians are usually good for referrals.

I worked with one woman in an assisted living apartment who kept a small, nippy, yappy dog. (I love dogs, but this one tried my patience.) The facility threatened to throw her out when the dog bit the postman. I promised the facility we would bring in a dog walker and trainer to rectify the situation. The deal worked out beautifully. The senior stayed in the apartment with her dog, and we were able eventually to eliminate the dog trainer's visits.

HAIRDRESSERS

Often a beloved hairdresser will come to the home of a long-standing client. If not, most beauty shops know of hairdressers who will make house calls for a reasonable fee. Hairdressing is one area where keeping up appearances counts, and can be essential to helping a senior maintain her self-image.

PRIVATE TRAINERS

Sometimes a senior needs additional conditioning after physical therapy formally ends. Ask around for referrals, especially at gyms, physical therapy centers and spas. Some physical therapists at home care agencies moonlight on the side.

MUSIC THERAPISTS

Music therapy is easy to overlook, but often surprisingly valuable. My daughter, now a professional harpist, often accompanied me to a client's home or assisted living facility. When younger, she would get upset when seniors fell asleep while she played, but I assured her it was a great compliment as her music helped the seniors feel at peace and relax.

Of course, it's important to find music the client likes. I used to play the accordion, but found that some seniors were afraid of them. An elderly woman once told me about a musician who, as she put it, shoved an accordion in her husband's face, frightening him. After that, he was reluctant to have any music at all.

CHEFS

Private chefs and ready-to-eat food providers are proliferating. Both are good options for picky seniors. Private chefs will come to a senior's home and cook several meals at a time, many of which can be frozen to heat up later. Meal plan companies can also be used for short or extended periods. They deliver their food directly to homes, either in bulk or by the day or week, and cater to special diets like kosher and vegetarian.

I always discussed food allergies and likes and dislikes with clients and their families. Some seniors relished nouveau cuisine, though most preferred meatloaf and mashed potatoes. Meals-on-wheels type programs that deliver food directly to seniors generally serve mediocre to good food. They're great options for seniors happy with the types of foods they offer. However, many seniors are not, and finding a chef or providing more sophisticated and varied food choices can bring pleasure as well as nourishment to seniors whose worlds are becoming ever more constrained.

Part 4

~~~~~~

Tough Calls

"Old age isn't so bad when you consider the alternative."
— *Maurice Chevalier*

CHAPTER 15

Overcoming the Senior "NO!"

Unless you are among the small minority with a passive or cooperative parent who welcomes assistance, your attempts to help will be met with resistance, sometimes mild, often fierce. "NO!" your Dad or Mom will say:

- ❖ No, I don't want to talk about it.
- ❖ No, I don't need any help.
- ❖ No, you don't know more than I do.
- ❖ No, you can't do that to me.
- ❖ No, I won't spend money for unnecessary help. Besides, it's too expensive.
- ❖ And no, not you or the State will get me out of this home.

I have seen parents pull out all the stops, including telling lies and threatening to shut their children out of their lives if they don't back off — even when the parent's situation is dangerous and the adult child knows the parent needs help.

This is what I think of as *The Senior NO,* and, at least at first, it's effective to the point at which many would-be helpers give up. After all, as children we grew used to backing off when parents said no, and we were terrified of being disowned. As children, most of us were taught our parents, like other adults, made safe decisions. Parents are childhood's primal authority figures, only one step below God.

Yet seniors can become nasty and defensive when they feel threatened. I remember standing in the driveway of a lovely couple's home. They were distraught, trying to get a demented father into the car to go to a secured assisted living facility. The family had done everything it could to make the move for "Pops" comfortable. But Pops insisted his son only wanted to take his money and get him out of the way. The son was so upset by Pops' repeated accusation of theft that he became paralyzed, unable to do anything. And the daughter-in-law felt it was not her place to intervene.

I helped them get Pops to the facility, and stayed with Pops for hours, going over and over the reasons he was there. Nobody was stealing his money, I repeated, and he would be fine. By evening, he was eating with his new group, telling everyone his son was a wonderful boy, and that he really liked the food. Later that night, I reassured the son. Dementia can be ugly, I said, adding that Pops did not mean the things he'd said, and besides, he'd already forgotten the whole affair. Pops never brought it up again.

I usually hear first from a daughter or daughter-in-law. One daughter-in-law who called me in despair said her husband was being pushed out of his parents' lives, and he was not able to ask for help. Instead, the son felt that if he could be more loving and argue one more time with his parents, Lenny and Irene, the outcome would be different. But Irene suffered from severe dementia. She was refusing to shower and eating erratically, and her diabetes was out of control. Lenny, frail and ill but mentally capable, was refusing to see a doctor. He and Irene spent most days watching TV and drinking alcohol.

I called a family meeting for Lenny, Irene, the daughter-in-law that contacted me and other children, and walked into a shouting match. The family dynamics had deteriorated into a destructive negative loop. Lenny viciously attacked every suggestion, and Irene agreed with whatever her husband said. Soon, the siblings started squabbling over different ways to approach the situation, and the meeting degenerated into a free for all.

I knew I would have to take command, and quickly, to have any hope of turning things around. First, I asked everyone to "zip it," in as light a tone of voice as I could muster. Then I listened, one by one, to each family member's concerns. I had to ask Lenny and Irene to zip it several times before they had their turns. Lenny was genuinely surprised to realize that everyone else could see what was going on with him and Irene. Once he did, he became very quiet.

I summarized everyone's issues, then discussed them with Lenny in front of the group. I did not hesitate, stutter or appear indecisive. I laid out the facts and the dangers, explaining to the couple what could happen if they refused to cooperate with their family and accept some level of home care. I also told Lenny about adult protective services — that they have the authority to come into an unsafe home and make it safe as they see fit, which could mean moving Irene out, and upsetting the plan to keep both of them at home. I did not threaten to call protective services, but pointed out their situation was so unsafe it was likely to be noticed by neighbors or Irene's doctor, any of whom might, on their own, call protective services.

I offered to bring in aides for a few hours a day, morning and evening at first, to cover meals and help care for Irene. This would give them needed structure and oversight, I explained, but also some privacy. Lenny accepted this, and I gradually increased the aides' hours as they became used to the arrangement.

Lenny and I eventually developed a close friendship. I loved to visit them; he would joke about what a horrible nag I was, but always with a twinkle in his eye. Lenny and Irene were able to continue living at home. And the family went back to visiting their parents without constantly worrying about medications, safety, and the threat of another crisis.

By the time some families find the will to break through a senior's resistance, a serious crisis may already be underway. As a result, I've learned the hard way that the longer a family or a caregiver waits to intervene or make a decision, the fewer resources and choices either ends up with. Consider falls: at least two dozen seniors have told me there was no way they could fall. Of course, quite a few did.

Ann was a spry senior who took pride in her appearance and her friends. She was unaware many friends had actually abandoned her because her ramblings and emotional outbursts confused them. I initially arranged to put care in her home. However, Ann became unstable on her feet, and her home was old, with several levels, rugs, no railings, and many places where she might fall. I felt Ann needed to be in a safer environment.

Ann adamantly refused to go anywhere — until her hip broke. We don't know if she fell and broke the hip or it broke on its own, causing Ann to fall. The result, either way, was the same — hip surgery and a long rehabilitation. Fortunately, Ann was able to walk again with a walker. But she did her walking in an assisted living facility, where she made friends and was able to revive some of the relationships she had lost. She was in the dementia part of the facility, but it included open areas, activities geared to her abilities, and many opportunities to socialize.

In dealing with seniors, it's important to examine the ways you can create success. This often means not only bringing in care, but changing the senior's environment by moving furniture, redoing bathrooms, turning a ground floor room into a bedroom, or just moving to a safer, more suitable home or apartment. But always remember to keep familiar items around.

Trips to emergency rooms and surgeries, and all the consequences that follow can change a family's life forever. Not everything is preventable, but many things are. It's vital to try and look below the surface of an aging parent's living arrangements. Too often, parents are able to convince children and others that everything is fine when it's not. Mom forgets to mention she fell down the stairs or can't figure out how to make a sandwich. Perhaps you sense all is not fine, but the prospect of their resistance undermines your intentions.

GETTING PAST NO

How do you get past *The Senior NO* to make something happen? Start by looking at the problem from your parent's perspective, and allow him to express his feelings. Underneath a senior's apparent anger, he is afraid and uncertain. Ceding you control, he fears, will permit you to do something he doesn't want and thinks he doesn't need. I often acknowledge this by realizing that, given the same circumstances, I would feel the same way.

Recognize that in the absence of anyone else, you need to take command. Be a leader, become empowered. Don't hesitate. If you're not sure what's going on, find a care manager and have an assessment made of the situation. Whether out of fear, habit, denial, dementia or just lousy judgment, your parents may have backed themselves into a corner. And because they know how to push you back better than anyone, their resistance will loom larger than it actually is.

Keep moving forward in a kind but firm and persistent manner. If an assessment reveals help is necessary, you must make it happen. Since solutions are not always easy or quick, be prepared to dig in and show a measure of patience.

When a parent realizes he cannot push you away, he will sometimes reluctantly listen. If such an opening presents itself, seize it. Persuasion is your first and best strategy. Tell the senior you know he doesn't like your meddling, but you want him to stay safe, and have his best interests in mind. Gift-wrap, if needed, your arguments: say you can work together as a team to make his life better.

Speak in a voice that's warm but decisive. Try to avoid getting off topic, especially if it leads to further disagreements. Stay focused, mention what you've noticed, and express your concern. Explain what you think should be discussed regarding help. Engage your parent's help as much as you can in keeping him safe, preferably at home. If you have a care manager, she can handle some of this, but you must be engaged as well. And when care or change is introduced, be there to ease it in place.

It often helps to start slowly. For example, tell the senior a "house-keeper" will be coming in a few hours a week just to help with laundry, cooking and similar chores. Begin by bringing in the home care only three times a week for two or three hours each time, gradually adding hours and days — and maybe a nurse to fill pill planners — as the senior becomes used to the assistance, and until he is being cared for properly.

THE TWO-MONTH SOLUTION

One of my most effective solutions is one of the simplest. I like to suggest to a senior that we try something for just two months, then reconsider. This can cover changing a schedule, bringing in home care or moving to a facility. It works like magic.

The senior feels he is not completely giving in. I feel the same, and the two-month period can provide needed information and care. I promise that at the end of two months, we will discuss the situation, whatever it is, with all concerned, and re-evaluate. At the end of the two months (less, if care uncovers additional issues), most seniors have accommodated themselves to the new assistance or circumstances and are actually grateful. If not, I tweak the plan for another two months. Many seniors forget there ever was an issue.

Ellen was a sweet elderly lady afflicted with dementia. And she was stubborn. For three solid hours, I passionately tried to convince her she needed to move into an assisted living dementia facility. She could no longer stay at home, even with help. But Ellen did not want to go. She said she had the right to live in a messy house and eat poorly, which was true.

But Ellen was not able to feed herself, and was wandering lost around the neighborhood. The family had exhausted itself trying to bring help into the house, but it wasn't working. Her house was set up for her to fail, and there was no way to make it safe. Ellen needed to live in a structured environment to succeed. But she had just enough logic left to argue with me.

I did not want to call protective services or have her daughter conserve her, giving her the legal authority to make Ellen's decisions for her. Finally, I decided to take charge and simply took Ellen to the facility — to which she agreed to go only if we revisited the issue again in two months. We did, but by then she had forgotten there had even been an argument. Ellen settled in and did fine. The two-month solution helped us scale and overcome the wall of her NO.

In fact, I would go so far as to recommend approaching almost every change as temporary, even if you are not sure. This makes it less scary for the senior, and you can always later make changes as needed.

If a situation is seriously dangerous — such as with seniors who leave the stove on or are hurting someone or themselves — you must act quickly, even if you have to remove the senior from the situation. If you are concerned about being considered abusive or your parent is threatening to call the police, you can always call adult protective services and explain what you are doing.

Or call an attorney or a care manager. Either can help with these kinds of decisions. Sometimes a senior is so impaired the court must conserve him and have someone else manage his life, but this is not often necessary. The bottom line is that if a parent is failing, it is often up to you to bring in the cavalry, and make the decisions you and others agree will improve the circumstances of your parent's life.

I had a client who was living with his demented wife in an assisted living facility. Ed was free to come and go, as he wasn't showing any signs of dementia when they moved in. However, as time went on, Ed began feeding his wife dangerous medications, spending large sums of money, and driving when not allowed. He was also becoming belligerent. After months of observation, tests, and medication trials, Ed's doctor, the family, the staff of the facility and I all agreed Ed would probably need to be conserved.

This meant his car would be taken away, he would no longer be allowed access to medication, an attorney would keep track of his money and give Ed what he needed, and Ed, like his wife, would have to obey the facility's rules. We tried many times and in many different ways to persuade him to follow the rules, but his judgment had grown so impaired, he was unable to do so. He was finally conserved, and life for him and his wife improved immensely. I don't ever like to have someone conserved, but if you run out of all other options, consider it.

THE BIG GUILT

It is common in dealing with aging parents to feel denial, resentment, fear, grief, anxiety, intimations of mortality, anger, and/or abandonment — and the biggest emotion of all, guilt. I certainly felt many of these emotions in dealing with my dad, and I have witnessed years of pent-up emotions tumbling out from others. If you are pushing a parent into something necessary and know his quality of life is at stake, no matter how better the change, guilt seems to follow.

I recently asked several family members I've worked with what they remember feeling. Guilt was the first emotion many mentioned. Even though they knew there were no choices other than those made to overcome their parents' resistance, they still felt guilty about making them.

On the other hand, once a decision is made and a plan is in place, you will often experience feelings of relief, empowerment and hope, and improved relationships with your parent and family members. Of course, guilt and other doubts may still creep in, but you will know you have done the best that could be done, and the right thing to have done.

Don't let your own fears and emotions stop you when a failing senior resists necessary care. If you cannot get past your emotions or a bitter, unworkable relationship with your parent, bring in professional help. Obtain counseling if you need it, go to a support group for caregivers, ask for help from family and friends, turn the case over to a care manager. But every senior, whether the greatest in the world or a nasty drunk, deserves kindness, mercy, and as safe and dignified a life as possible.

CHAPTER 16

Taking the Car and
Other Special Issues

Aging is an obstacle course strewn with unexpected problems, many difficult to face, many that fly in the face of logic, and many that can make the best plans fail. Though they are not unique, these problems often defy simple solutions. To succeed, you may have to come at a problem from different angles, be very patient, and know when to seek help. Here are a few of the thorny issues the children of aging parents can expect to confront, and some ideas for doing so.

How Do I know It's Time to Take Away My Mother's or Father's Driver's License? And How Do I Do It?

If you suspect a problem with driving, there probably is one. Assess the situation to confirm your suspicion. Have there been any explained or unexplained accidents recently? Is the car exhibiting fresh dents or scuffs? Go for a drive with your parent and see how he handles intersections, quick decisions and stoplights. Try it at night as well. Does he tend to confine his driving to one small area? Has he gotten lost? Drive behind him and observe.

If you think a license should be taken away, don't chicken out. This is a huge deal, but the senior's self-esteem can be rebuilt and is less important than his safety and the safety of others on the road. First, try persuasion. Explain that times have changed, that today's roads are filled with traffic and crazy drivers, that it's easier not to drive, and less costly than maintaining a car that's being used less and less.

Tell him he should not be driving given the many medications he's taking. Say, truthfully, you're concerned about his safety on the road. If logic doesn't work, tell him that if he gets into an accident and his medical files are pulled, he could lose his home if his insurance won't cover the accident, which it may not.

Do not plead or bargain. If you're convinced the senior should no longer drive, the bottom line must be no car. Period. If you are still talking to a brick wall, call your State's Department of Motor Vehicles (DMV) or visit its website. All DMVs have medical oversight departments that deal with issues involving elderly drivers, dementia and other problems. They will provide information on the form and procedure for having someone's license suspended or rescinded. It usually requires a doctor's statement that the person should not drive. If your parent's primary doctor declines to send one, try a specialist. If you get nowhere, find out if the DMV has a form that a concerned citizen, like yourself, can fill out and submit. Some States give seniors the option of being tested by the DMV or a contracted program, like Easter Seals. Some States simply cancel a senior's license and notify him by mail.

I remember one client with dementia who was hallucinating about ocean liners in his front yard. I physically took his license away and hid it in a drawer. He was fine with that. However, one of his daughters took him to a program to clear him for driving. It so happened he enjoyed an unusually lucid two hours during this outing and passed the test. After that, I never again trusted the testing.

Often, I would go to a DMV and get its handbook of driving and traffic rules. Then I would give it to a senior and tell him he needed to study it before taking a driving test. Of course, he complained, as they all did. But the handbook proved so daunting I never had a senior question me further about taking a driving test.

If a senior insists on driving, test or no test, and is hiding the car keys or lying about using the car, you are left with two commando options. One is to move the car to a friend's house or somewhere else for a few weeks or months, and tell the senior his car is being worked on. The longer you wait it out, the more his desire to drive, and the force of his habit, will wane. The other option is to visit a local police station or department and explain the situation. The police can actually be very helpful. I have known them to follow seniors and take their licenses at the first signs of anything amiss. You will feel guilty, but you will feel worse if your parent accidentally drives into a storefront.

Do not pull a car's wires or plugs. Resourceful seniors will call the AAA or a repair shop and have the car fixed. Even a frail woman can ask her neighbor to look at her car, and soon find herself driving again.

Taking a car away may be hard, but dealing with what could otherwise easily happen is much harder. To compensate for the car's loss, look into whether your town has senior vans of some sort, hire a driver through a healthcare agency or find volunteers. After a while, all of my seniors came to enjoy being driven around. Most liked the attention, and were relieved they no longer had to cope with the stress of driving, parking and maintaining the car. If a family member can't handle the situation, immediately involve a GCM.

WHAT IF A PARENT IS DRINKING EXCESSIVELY?

This is a difficult situation because someone used to drinking every day will want, and may feel compelled, to continue the habit. I have had many clients with dementia who had been alcoholics for decades. I had one who sipped several drinks a night because he forgot how much he was drinking, and others whose drinking, in my opinion, fueled their dementia.

When approaching a drinking parent, start with logic. Tell him such things as:

- ❖ You're taking too many medications to risk mixing them with alcohol.
- ❖ The doctor says you can't drink. (Ask the doctor to back you up.)
- ❖ You might fall and break a hip or a leg, and become disabled.
- ❖ You may decide to cook, drive or do something else potentially dangerous while your judgment is impaired.

Such statements usually didn't work in my own experience, compelling me to assign an aide at night to fix dinners and try to limit the alcohol intake; for example, by hiding the bottle after an evening's initial drink. I have removed alcohol from homes, rationed alcohol, detoxed seniors, but only had one client realize she could call a liquor store and ask it to deliver. Sometimes an aide's presence in the evening helps the family realize just how much the senior is drinking, a fact both the family and the doctor should know.

One client with dementia had a husband who was caring for her, but also drinking himself to oblivion every night. I sent an aide in chiefly to keep an eye on the client while her husband drank. This turned out to be a good idea, as the husband hurt himself one night and the aide called for help. Another client turned mean when he drank and verbally tormented his demented wife. I threatened to call in protective services, and he cut back on the drinking. I also put an aide in the house to make sure the drinking stayed cut back. If a parent is living with another family member who is drinking and being abusive, calling protective services becomes a must unless the drinker can be reasoned with and his drinking reduced.

Excessive drinking simply cannot be tolerated. Too many seniors fall in their homes and break hips or other bones, or die. Drinkers fall more often. Despite this, some seniors will continue to drink, and there is little to do but put in place the safety measures noted above and make sure key family members and doctors understand the situation.

If a senior is hospitalized, let the staff know he drinks, and how much. Don't assume the staff will always pick it up. They won't, and a senior accustomed to alcohol cannot stop drinking immediately without medical supervision. Delirium tremens, the DTs, do happen and are no joke. They are always serious and can be life-threatening. I have known hospitalized seniors used to sneaking alcohol who endured the DTs because nobody alerted the staff.

WHAT IF YOU SUSPECT A PARENT IS BEING NEGLECTED OR ABUSED?

Always take suspicions of neglect or abuse seriously. Seniors do not usually tell anyone because they're afraid the abusers may hurt them or they won't be believed. Look for bruises, cuts and changes in behavior. Think about whether the senior is more withdrawn or quiet or acting strangely around a family member or caregiver.

Seniors should not be yelled at, shoved, left uncomfortable, hurt in any way or left alone if not safe. Neglect, after all, is just another form of abuse. If someone supposedly caring for a senior is not keeping the senior safe, fed and comfortable, there is a problem. It may be self-neglect, but if nobody steps up to correct the situation, protective services may need to intervene.

When I suspected abuse or neglect and questions and attempts at support failed to elicit any information, I often resorted to spying and surprise. I would visit the client's house at all times of the day or night, for example, without calling ahead. Approaching the home, I would look and listen for what was going on inside, then pop in and assess the reaction when I appeared. Was the caregiver nervous? Was the senior dressed appropriately? Or did he look relieved? If you have suspicions, your GCM should call protective services and discuss your concerns. They should work with you to find out what is going on.

WHAT IF THE ADULT CHILDREN ARE SQUABBLING?

For a variety of reasons, siblings can turn antagonistic when a parent is sick or dying. As a result, serious disagreements among family members are a huge problem. The disagreements tend to follow familiar patterns. Old resentments surface, and the primary caregiver becomes the target of verbal sniping ranging from annoying to downright mean. I have witnessed "loving" siblings tear each other apart because the primary caregiver needed help, and the other siblings were not used to doing any work.

It is not uncommon for a local daughter or son who is caring for a parent to be visited by out-of-state siblings who have arrived for a visit. They may berate the local sibling, while offering their own solutions, which usually prove unworkable. The sibling in the trenches doing the hardest work gets questions rather than support. Nor is it uncommon in the presence of a declining parent for family members to curry favor, manipulate or act badly.

During one such instance in my practice, the primary caregiver started to retreat into a fog of guilt and self-doubt. I stated the obvious — that she had been on the front lines all along, and her brothers and sisters did not want to take on any responsibilities for themselves. They only wanted their sister to continue to bear the burden and continue doing the work she always had. When the caregiver finally learned to say "no" and got her siblings to help, the family calmed down and proceeded to do what was needed.

A family member taking a lead role and delegating certain duties to others can usually resolve minor issues. If the squabbling is really bad, a GCM can come in and moderate. Some eldercare specialists, mostly attorneys, offer family mediation services. This was a large part of my practice, in fact. I often held family meetings to go over everyone's concerns and complaints, and then, with their input acknowledged, moved toward solutions. Sometimes I had to be tough, but mediation, with an outsider as the mediator, was always a practical option.

What If a Parent Needs Immediate Help, and There's No Money?

Several options are available, but they depend on what a senior needs, the urgency of the problem, and the skill of the family or its GCM in shaking the benefits tree. You can look into State programs, which are income and asset based, or seek State help with a Medicaid application. If the senior is living at home and care needs to come in, a reverse mortgage can be a practical way to raise funds, bearing in mind the field is riddled with scammers and a lawyer should review any agreement.

Veteran benefits, another process requiring applications and patience, may be available. Alternatively, family members may need to help with their own funds, and with little or no expectation of being repaid.

What If My Father or Mother Won't Accept a Caregiver of Color, or Someone Obese?

I always tried to accommodate a senior's wishes as much as possible, because if I assigned an aide I knew would cause a problem, it would be hard on the aide as well as the senior. This was not always fair to the aide, but unavoidable. Many older seniors no longer even understand the issue, make unintentionally racist remarks and insult caregivers horribly.

One of my clients actually talked about lynching black people, in front of his black aide no less. When I opened my mouth to tell him he was being inappropriate, he told me no one could ever hang me as I would break the tree (I was overweight at the time). That stung.

Surprisingly, seniors who fight the hardest against accepting particular aides often develop close bonds with them. I have witnessed many happy turnarounds, including one involving the client who targeted his aide's color and my weight. He and his African-American caregiver became friends, proving there's always room for growth.

WHAT IF I PROMISED NEVER TO PUT MY MOTHER OR FATHER IN A NURSING HOME?

First of all, don't ever promise such a thing. When a senior can no longer stay at home — for whatever reason: behavior, wandering, lack of funds or a condition needing skilled care — you will not want to feel guilty for having to break that promise.

If you have already made the promise, and it's too late, just do your best. If the move is to assisted living, emphasize to the senior that he'll be going to an apartment, not a nursing home. If a nursing home is actually needed and there is no alternative, understand that you did not know what you were promising. Do not beat yourself up. Your father or mother will still need your care and concern. Paralysis and regret help no one, you included.

WHAT IF MY PARENT IS FROM ANOTHER CULTURE AND DOESN'T TRUST ANYONE?

Usually, the immediate family of a parent from another country speaks the senior's language, and one of the children serves as the liaison between the senior and the rest of the world. But healthcare professionals may frighten a senior who speaks little or no English, provoking a kind of fear that only intensifies with dementia. If this sounds like your parent, look for one of the many facilities or home care agencies that have people from other cultures who can act as translators. Just hearing a native language from an outsider can calm a nervous senior.

If your parent's language is not one common in your area, you may have to seek out a translator through an online search for translators or churches, schools and groups in an area that embrace that particular culture and language. I had a very difficult case in which a daughter was caring for her foreign-born parents. She spoke their language, but they wouldn't listen to her because she was the daughter. And they wouldn't listen to any of the healthcare professionals because they only spoke English. Finally, I found a social worker at a local nursing home who spoke the seniors' language, and was able to convince the parents to trust us enough to bring help in.

How Do I Handle My Parent Having a Relationship at a Facility?

While this may seem unlikely, it happens, especially in facilities oriented toward clients with memory loss. If your dad's a widower and lonely, sometimes it's helpful for him to bond with another person, even of the other sex. He may think she's his wife or daughter, and may eat or converse with her. If this is where it ends, be happy the seniors can enjoy each other's company and have something upon which to build a social structure.

But problems can develop if relationships go beyond this level. I worked with a daughter who had both parents in an assisted living memory-care facility. While the wife was temporarily in a hospital, the demented husband — call him Jerry — was pining for her. He had no idea how long she'd been away (a couple weeks), and wasn't sure if she was coming back. At this point of maximum vulnerability, a very aggressive female resident decided she was Jerry's wife and pushed his family and everyone else away.

One day, they were found naked in a room. Meanwhile, Jerry's actual wife died. This left his daughter to deal with the death of a parent and the craziness going on with another woman taking advantage of her father. The staff tried to redirect the woman, but she was determined to treat her imagined husband as hers. Jerry was polite, but unsure about what was going on.

Such behavior may also have legal ramifications, depending on the State and the feelings of those involved. To participate in sexual acts, a person, male or female, must be able to give consent. With one or two demented individuals, consent becomes a very gray concept. Showing that even one senior's judgment is impaired can create the possibility of a non-consenting partner.

When assisted living was new and I raised questions about consent to my superiors, they said sexual relations between residents with dementia could be tolerated only if the children gave consent. I doubted the validity of this then and still do. If a genuine relationship develops between seniors in assisted living, the appropriate approach is to talk to the families, the facility, even an attorney, to make sure nobody is getting hurt.

Be aware also of the possibility of a romantic interest pursued for purposes of marriage or money from the other senior. In my experience, assisted-living affairs almost always involved a woman pursuing some unsuspecting guy. If you are uncomfortable with anything like this going on in a facility, alert the staff immediately in writing. Give them a chance to resolve the situation, even to the point of hiring an extra aide to make sure nothing untoward happens.

If the facility cannot or does not resolve the situation, you may need to move your parent to another facility. Don't just hope the problem will go away. The senior's safety, as always, should be paramount.

How Do I Know Hospice is Needed? And What Do I Tell My Mother or Father?

If you think a senior has only six to twelve months to live and is uncomfortable, you or your GCM can contact a hospice agency and ask it to do an evaluation. You can also bring it up with your parent's doctor. If the parent does not want to talk about death, tell him a special group of nurses and other people will be coming in to help.

Hospice workers have training and medications designed for palliative care, or making a person more comfortable as the end nears, even before an actual hospice intervention. Hospice service needs to be ordered by an M.D. Usually, the family doctor will do it. At this point, you can tell the hospice people how you would like them to present to the senior what they are doing.

Typically, a hospice nurse will come out to the home, perform an intake, and decide if the hospice's criteria are met. If so, Medicare covers most of the care, allowing the agency to immediately bring in help, equipment and medications.

A great many agencies provide hospice care, and the senior's doctor should know which is best in your area. If not, call a GCM or ask around. Hospices with physical facilities generally don't accept patients until they are close to death or need pain control. Some nursing homes also designate areas or floors as hospices, and move patients there when the time comes.

CHAPTER 17

You, the Person in Charge

Many adult children are already tired by the time they contact me, worn down by the difficult situations they have been handling. Usually, there has been a crisis, and delay has limited their options. As the nature of the crisis becomes clear, the seniors' children find themselves growing increasingly desperate and, often, grasping at whatever help is available, even though it may have negative consequences down the road.

It is far better to set up short and long term plans before a crisis breaks. Of course, no one can anticipate or plan for everything, so even the best-laid plans "aft gang agley," as Robert Burns famously wrote. But almost any plan is better than none, and the effort to create one will alert you to much you did not know before.

Let's be honest; stepping into a parental-style role with your own parent can be sad and depressing. But faced with an unsafe situation, you must do something. And once a process begins, a better relationship with your parent may result. He will be safer and happier, and you can take a breath and feel comforted by knowing you have done all you can.

In the short term, a parent's safety and comfort should be the paramount objectives. In the long term, quality of life can play a larger role. Once you start doing anything, many parents will interpret it as meddling and resist. Be prepared for this reaction. However difficult, stay strong, and don't back down. You can listen and be supportive, but don't be bullied or unduly put off by a senior's resistance.

If you address your concerns frankly and bring in help, the help will free you to shape a better relationship with your parent. Instead of worrying whether he's eating enough or taking his pills, you can let someone else do that (or whatever is needed), and spend quality time with him, visiting and sharing something mutually enjoyable.

PRIORITIZE

As in any planning process, step one is to sort out the priorities. Ask whether:

- ❖ You need immediate help or have some time to look around.
- ❖ There is a crisis.
- ❖ The senior can't be alone.
- ❖ You need a care manager or care from an agency.
- ❖ The senior's home situation is becoming inappropriate.

If the answers are yes, don't immediately jump to a placement option — unless there are pressing issues like wandering or resistance to necessary care, in other words, something that requires a new environment with more structure and predictability. This is usually a hard call. Often, it comes after home care has already been tried and the care better illuminates the actual situation, making you realize the senior's home has become too unsafe for his continued residence.

Once, I had a client with dementia who lived alone with her dog. She began to think the dog was her late husband and didn't understand why he spent so much time on the floor. Many a time she almost tripped over the dog. At the same time, she grew afraid to be alone and was starting to wander. Home care was not enough to significantly help, so she was moved to an assisted living dementia facility. She thrived, and felt relieved to have the company of others.

Never assume you know what any senior is thinking. No one knows with certainty what's in the mind of someone with cognitive issues. He could be living in a different reality, worried about strange things, and unable to express any of it. Having a lot of time alone, seniors sometimes start imagining new worlds, which can be very scary. Two separate clients, already in dementia facilities, tried on separate occasions to throw chairs out the windows to help the people escape from "something." We never found out what.

As you work toward a plan, use the facts, your gut, the available options and support, and whether something needs to be done immediately or just soon, allowing you more time to explore resources and options. In planning for a senior, you'll find most short-term issues revolve around safety and comfort.

Safety First

Above all, you'll want your parent to be safe. Consider his physical, psychological, memory and other mental issues. Can he get hurt physically? Are there falling issues? Go over his house and see what he's doing, especially at night.

Does your parent need watching all the time? Or is it enough to have someone come in for chores like housekeeping, medications or meals? I always prefer keeping a senior at home and bringing in care as needed. But if a house is unsafe for the senior, another location may be indicated. If dementia is causing your parent to wander, cook in the middle of the night or exhibit other warning signs (see Chapter 2), someone may need to check in frequently, spend the night or stay around the clock.

Emergency pendants can be useful. However, many seniors, especially with dementia, cannot remember how to use them. Medications need to be monitored, and many seniors often don't eat unless someone prepares their food.

Comfort Next

What does quality of life mean in the context of a senior in decline? Here are some parameters: Seniors should be able to see and hear as well as they are able. They should be able to socialize, not suffer from pain, feel safe from abuse and neglect, sleep in comfortable beds, and eat healthful food. They should be among their own possessions, enjoy the respect of attendants, and not worry about their bills being paid. Stress should be minimized, and they should be able to go out shopping if capable of doing so, visit with friends, and continue to do whatever makes them feel good.

Once these quality-of-life elements are secured to the extent possible, you can focus on the longer term. Finances will dictate a great deal of what can be done, so this is a time to look at State programs, solicit advice from an eldercare attorney, and decide if a parent can stay at home with or without care (and how much). It's also a time to figure out what devices may be helpful, and how much other family members will contribute to the workload and financing. Evaluate these activities by looking ahead in time frames ranging from two-to-six months in the future to one year, two years, and so on.

WAYS TO BRING IN HELP

Almost every senior I have dealt with feels he is fine, and doesn't need anything. But if your parent's situation has become urgent, you will have to act and, usually, act quickly. Here are your primary options:

- ❖ Stay with your parent yourself — rotating, if possible, with family and friends — until more structured assistance can be arranged.
- ❖ Contact a Geriatric Care Manager and have her recommend care. Most GCMs can perform assessments on short notice.
- ❖ Call and interview home care and/or visiting nurse agencies to determine their prices, the types of care they provide, and if they offer what you need. Make sure they can cover all necessary shifts. Their care can often be covered by Medicare, but not for long periods.
- ❖ Call a live-in agency if needed.
- ❖ Consider assisted living, especially facilities equipped for dementia care if the senior is having issues at home. Some facilities offer emergency respites, allowing you to pay by the day until you can better sort things out.
- ❖ If your parent is resisting and complaining about every suggestion, and the situation is urgent, ignore his squawking and just bring in the help. Safety trumps defiance.
- ❖ In the event of a serious medical crisis, there is always the emergency room.

If you need money quickly and have no other front-line financial resources, consider a reverse mortgage on the senior's home or condo. But be careful, the field is rife with ruinous but seductive-sounding deals.

Alternatively, borrow from family members on a short-term basis until their funds can be reimbursed.

If you have the luxury of time, you can perform these activities at a more leisurely pace, adding more as you progress.

COVER THE BASES

As we've seen, caring for a senior is a big job. It requires certain levels of personal authority and responsibility, a high level of attentiveness, and specialized documents, services and equipment. Since every case varies in its particulars, so will your needs. Here are some of the key things you're likely to need, or want, to properly fill out your senior care toolkit:

Documents

❖ Set up and maintain a **medical notebook** detailing the senior's insurance information and medical history as well as current conditions, medications, doctors and lab reports. Include everything pertinent to his care. Take it with you to all appointments and keep it updated.

❖ Obtain a **Power of Attorney** for personal and financial issues and keep several copies, as you will likely need to present one to different agencies or individuals.

❖ Make sure someone is getting and paying the senior's bills.

❖ Compose a sheet of paper listing **contact information and the senior's conditions and medications.** Post a copy on your fridge and the senior's. Hand it to emergency responders coming to the house or grab it if you're going to the ER.

❖ **Do Not Resuscitate** (DNR) and CPR instructions: decide in advance of needing them what they will be should your parent become unresponsive. They are more complicated than you may realize so you will want to think about them, and consult with your parent, if he is capable of understanding, and other family members. Act similarly for any other medical wishes the senior has. If you are unwilling or unable to bear this responsibility, consider having a healthcare agent, with a Power of Attorney, appointed specifically to make sure the senior's health wishes are carried out as instructed.

Be aware that if there are no directives, responders and doctors will do everything they can to maintain life, including installing a ventilator and a feeding tube. And once such devices are running, it becomes much harder to have them removed.

Speak with your parent about what is happening and involve him to the extent he can handle it. In particular, discuss plans with your parent once a crisis is averted, and reassure him you are trying to keep him safe and happy.

❖ **Prescriptions** for equipment or devices: some may be covered by Medicare, but always check first with a doctor or equipment provider as the scripts have to be written in a certain way to qualify.

Services

❖ **Meals on Wheels:** Most towns have a program for seniors that delivers one or more meals on all or most days.

❖ Consider **home delivery of groceries** by stores or online delivery services like FreshDirect, Peapod and NetGrocer.

❖ **Physical Therapy:** Medicare often covers a physical therapist for home visits to help a senior, and also to adapt his home for easier, safer use. Private physical therapists, often moonlighting agency therapists, are also available.

❖ Professional **organizers** are individuals and agencies that help seniors sort out what is important to keep and what is best disposed of. Some also sell antiques, and make spaces safer.

❖ **Pharmacies** will often package medication doses in packets to be taken at specific times or place pills in a weekly planner. However, a senior using this service may still need help opening the planner and taking the medications.

Equipment

❖ Pill planners

❖ A lockable box to hold pill planners if the senior is confusing the dosages and medication times. In such cases, a caregiver will open the locked box and supervise medication times.

- ❖ A shower or bath seat
- ❖ A raised toilet seat
- ❖ A commode by the bed if the bathroom is too far for the senior to handle.
- ❖ One or more grab bars
- ❖ A cane or a walker
- ❖ One or two wheelchairs (a light model for transportation, and a sturdier one for home use)
- ❖ An emergency button for the senior to push for help (this will entail monthly service and possible other costs)
- ❖ Bedrails (though a potential hazard if the senior is likely to try to climb over them)
- ❖ A lift chair recliner or reclining lift chair: I have had many clients spend considerable time, and even sleep, in them. Medicare will pay part of the cost, since the chairs include motors that lift the seats up. My father fought against one for several years. After he finally agreed, he lived in it most of the time.
- ❖ Cushions for skin protection.
- ❖ A chair lift for stairs.
- ❖ A baby monitor is one of the best ways to keep track of a senior, especially at night. Some models include video cameras.
- ❖ Cameras to check on caregivers, or the senior.

WILL LIFE EVER BE THE SAME?

In caring for a senior, starting is often the hardest part. The next hardest is surviving the early stages when things seem to get worse before they get better. Stay focused, firm, loving and flexible. While individuals have the right to act stupidly, seniors too often confuse this with the ability to stay safe. As your senior care progresses, be prepared to also examine yourself, especially in the presence of guilt, old feelings, and other issues that may rise up from your childhood.

Above all, move ahead positively and ask for help when you need it. More help is available than you likely realize, as plenty of our generation's members are dealing with eldercare issues. Support groups and newsletters for seniors, family members, and caregivers are everywhere. But the vast majority are local and can best be found by asking doctors, home care agencies, nursing homes and by just searching on the Internet.

Even most of my own cases, complicated and trying in the beginning, only seemed to grow more difficult as the resistance to change — from everyone — emerged and asserted itself. However, as time moved on, seniors and family members usually embraced the changes they first resisted and grew relieved that something positive was being done.

Senior care can be a lonely undertaking, taking charge can be daunting, right and wrong can appear to blur, and you may find yourself feeling angry, remorseful, guilty, unsettled or depressed. Don't keep these feelings or reactions to yourself. Seek help in dealing with them, such as therapy and support from friends and others who have been through what you're experiencing. Support groups, now increasingly numerous, can be an oasis for a caregiver.

The bottom line is that whatever the situation, you can tackle it. Take the first step, try not to be afraid, and keep moving forward.

Epilogue

After Dad died, my sister Peach decided to hold a viewing of his body. I was opposed as Dad had outlived all his friends and we in the family had been with Dad at the end to send him off with love.

However, Peach felt the terrible way he looked after dying — his "death mask" wore a waxy face with a gaping mouth — was too much for her to handle as a last memory. She wanted to see and remember him outfitted once more wearing his ham radio shirt with his usual suspenders and a peaceful expression gracing his features.

When the day of the viewing came, I decided to stay with Dad because I did not want him left alone in the room. I knew this was a little crazy, especially since I felt his spirit was gone. But I loved my sister, and if the viewing would help give her some peace, sitting by his body was the least I could do, especially considering all the times Peach had been there for Dad when I could not.

As I walked into the viewing room that morning, I saw Dad bedecked in his favorite ham radio shirt and suspenders. His hair was slicked back with Brylcreem, which he always wore and which still gave off the distinctive smell we'd long grown used to. But Dad was also wearing bright pink lipstick. Horrified, I wiped it off, and was a little freaked out by how it felt to touch his body. And shocked, too, by my reaction, given the decades I'd been working as a professional nurse. I was also angry the funeral home hadn't done a better make-up job.

Enlisting some help, I propped up Dad's gigantic stuffed fish against a nearby wall, displayed a portrait of my parents on their wedding day, and had Fats Waller, Dad's favorite musician, playing in the background.

I spent the whole day there as people paraded in and out. Most had not known Dad, but wanted to pay their respects to the family. The experience felt so empty and weird that my niece, Jonette, and I began to tell each other every joke we could think of. Dad was a real jokester, and carried in his head a repertory of gags, many quite raunchy, on almost every subject.

By late afternoon, all four of my nieces and I were laughing so hard the funeral home staff must have thought we had lost our minds. But I still can't think of a better tribute to Dad than sitting around cracking each other up by telling his jokes. Just before the viewing ended, we stopped with the jokes. My sister Peach and her husband came in, and we all said our goodbyes. She had no idea what we had done to get through the day. I don't think Peach would have minded, but I knew the viewing was important to her, and I didn't want to appear inconsiderate.

It's been a while now since Dad passed away, yet I still sometimes pick up the phone to call him before remembering, sadly, he will not be there to answer my call at the other end. And I am reminded again, as so often in my life and work, that for those who are truly loved, not even death can fully sever the longest embrace.

Selected Resources

In this section is a brief list of websites offering valuable information about healthcare services and providers available to seniors and their families:

American Association of Retired Persons | www.aarp.org
AARP provides clear answers about healthcare and insurance (which it also sells) for seniors. The site also includes a wealth of information about government programs, especially Medicare, and is easier to navigate than government sites.

Alzheimer's Association | www.alz.org
This leading voluntary health organization for Alzheimer's care, support and research, offers a newsletter and considerable information about Alzheimer's disease and other forms of dementia.

Buck & Buck | www.buckandbuck.com
This site offers a collection of adaptive clothing and devices for seniors and others with disabling medical conditions. Items include clothing designed for ease of dressing, special shoes for those with edema, and extra-large socks.

Caregiver | www.caregiver.com
Today's Caregiver, an online version of the magazine for family and professional caregivers, includes many articles on caregiving, diseases and other medical conditions, special diets, cooking, and a finder for local support groups and other resources.

Drugs.Com | www.drugs.com
A quick, convenient, comprehensive source of information on medications, drug interactions, and pill identification marks, can be found on this site.

Eldercare Locator | www.eldercare.gov
A service of the U.S. Administration on Aging, *Eldercare Locator* connects individuals to community-based programs and services for older adults and their families. Although a bit overwhelming, it's a good place to start finding local resources.

Embracing Senior Care | www.embracingseniorcare.com
Barbara R. Hornby's website, focused on *Your Senior and You*, offers an engaging mix of in-depth information, articles, and opportunities for discussion and feedback about senior care and other issues facing the elderly and those looking after them.

FootSmart | www.FootSmart.com
FootSmart offers many types of comfortable shoes, reasonably-priced inserts and insoles, foot and toe protective products, and expandable slippers. The site also offers products and ideas for dealing with diabetic feet, bunions, hammertoes, calluses, heel pain and corns.

GoldViolin | www.goldviolin.com
GoldViolin offers a vast array of adaptive equipment and clothing with many interesting items, including some that blend well with furnishings.

Limbkeepers | www.limbkeepers.com
Limbkeepers, a new company, offers attractive sleeves to protect fragile skin on arms, legs and hands from abrasions, scrapes and bruising. Its non-compression knit sleeves are cushioned and come in a variety of colors.

Medicaid | www.medicaid.gov
The U.S. government site for the Medicaid program offers a wealth of information, including a finder for State Medicaid sites.

MedicAlert Foundation | www.medicalert.org
MedicAlert provides ID bracelets and cards with critical medical and contact information for caregivers or emergency first responders. This is a potential lifesaver for patients who have dementia or cannot speak for themselves. MedicAlert also operates a Safe Return program with the Alzheimer's Association (see www.alz.org for details) for patients who wander.

Medicare | www.medicare.gov
The U.S. government site for the Medicare program offers a vast repository of information about the program's coverage, costs and supplements. It includes online forms and information about claims and appeals, home care agencies, and the status of individual nursing homes. Note that each State also has its own Medicare site as rules vary widely.

National Association of Professional Geriatric Care Managers (NAPGCM) | www.caremanager.org
The site describes what GCMs do, and includes a finder to help users locate care managers in their areas as well as a directory with information about individual GCMs.

Philips Lifeline | www.lifelinesys.com
Philips Lifeline, a pioneer in the medical alert service industry, sells pendants and wrist buttons seniors can easily turn on to secure help in an emergency as well as Lifeline with AutoAlert, an automatic fall detection system that relies on a pendant.

A Place for Mom | www.aplaceformom.com
This service helps locate senior housing, assisted living and "memory care" facilities, and "senior living advisors" and includes useful articles about many aspects of senior life. Services are free to consumers, but be aware the site is compensated by facilities receiving successful referrals.

**Quality Homecare Products |
www.qualityhomecareproducts.com**
Quality Homecare Products specializes in the home delivery of
incontinence supplies, including adult diapers and disposable wipes.

Total Home Care Supplies | www.totalhomecaresupplies.com
Total Home Care Supplies offers a broad range of essential supplies,
from incontinence products and gloves to underpads, creams, catheters,
and ostomy and wound supplies.

Veterans Benefits Administration | www.benefits.va.gov
The U.S. government site for veterans' benefits, with explanations of
available benefits and how they work, is dense with information, and so
outside consultation with a specialist is suggested.

VITAS | www.vitas.com
VITAS Innovative Hospice Care provides a spectrum of services that
allow people to stay at home as they near the end, although Vitas also
offers facility-based hospice care. The company emphasizes comfort and
quality of life, and its personalized teams include nurses and aides.

Acknowledgements

I am grateful to the many people who have contributed to and supported me through the learning curve of senior care, and the additional learning curve required to write this book about my personal journey.

I want to thank my parents, Jack and Elaine Hachten, in particular, for loving and always believing in me, no matter what, and for encouraging me to think outside the box. My husband of almost 40 years, John Hornby, deserves a medal for putting up with my stepping off a cliff to start a business. He rearranged his life to accommodate my new schedule, contributed enormously to raising our children, and helped me with many technical issues. John's belief in me and his loving, unconditional devotion and support provided the foundation from which I was able bring my ideas to life.

My children, Elaine and Sena, deserve recognition for dealing with a confusing situation. I started my business partly so I could work around their schedules, but more often they worked around mine, which soon became 24/7, with telephones ringing at all hours and me, their mom, taking off for hours or days at a time to tend to needy clients and their families.

Peach, my sister, was there for Dad every day in his final years, and never asked for anything. Jonette, Peach's daughter, was also instrumental in Dad's care, and both encouraged me to write this book. Ron, Peach's husband, I thank for his kindness and patience in helping my dad at the end, especially in helping to get him the recliner he so came to value after years of resistance. I thank too my nieces, their families and my other family members for enriching Dad's life when it was most difficult by including him in family events.

Let me also acknowledge the family members, friends and co-workers who were extremely supportive as I struggled to translate my thoughts onto paper. They listened to my insecurities and doubts, lifted me up when needed and kept me on the right path. In particular, let me mention Stacey DeBruin, one of the best Care Managers I have ever known, for her astute counsel, support and advice about helping seniors and their families; and Shari Chan and Maureen Appi, fellow pioneers in care management, for helping me find the courage to keep moving forward at moments when I felt I could do no more.

The families I served deserve my thanks as well, for it was my efforts in their behalf that made me who I am, and fueled my passion to help the elderly. I feel like I am a part of each family I came to know, and will never forget the bonds we forged over the years. And to the aides, nurses, family members and other caregivers who with love and grace rolled up their sleeves to perform the thankless, often unpleasant, sometimes over-whelming tasks necessary to help vulnerable seniors — I applaud you.

I was fortunate to have had Stan Pinkwas as my editor. He pulled more out of me than I thought possible, tolerated my bad jokes, calmed my anxieties, and overcame my reluctance to write in a personal vein.

And if I am overlooking someone, know that in my heart you are acknowledged.

www.ingramcontent.com/pod-product-compliance
Lightning Source LLC
Chambersburg PA
CBHW072150270326
41931CB00010B/1946